40 DAYS TO
BETTER LIVING
OPTIMAL HEALTH

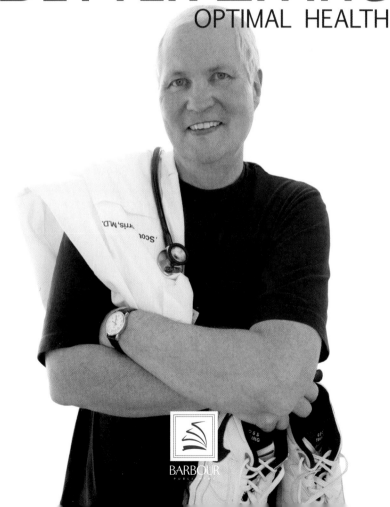

BARBOUR
PUBLISHING

Cover photography: Murray Riss Photography

Published by Barbour Publishing, Inc., P.O. Box 719, Uhrichsville, Ohio 44683
www.barbourbooks.com

Our mission is to publish and distribute inspirational products offering exceptional value and biblical encouragement to the masses.

 Member of the
Evangelical Christian
Publishers Association

Printed in the United States of America.

CONTENTS

Welcome,
From Dr. Scott Morris,
Founder of the Church Health Center

I first came to Memphis in 1986. I had no personal ties to Memphis and did not know anyone here. Having completed theological and medical education, I was determined to begin a health care ministry for the working poor. The next year, the doors of the Church Health Center opened with one doctor—me—and one nurse. We saw 12 patients the first day. Today we handle about 36,000 patient visits each year and 120,000 visits to our wellness facility. A staff of 250 people share a ministry of healing and wellness, and hundreds more volunteer time and services.

So what sets us apart from other community clinics around the country?

The Church Health Center is fundamentally about the church. We care for our patients without relying on government funds, because God calls the church to healing work. Jesus' life was about healing the whole person—body and spirit—and the church is Jesus in the world. His message is our message. His ministry is our ministry. Local congregations embrace this calling and help make our work possible.

More than two decades of caring for the working uninsured makes one thing plain: health care needs to change. In the years that the

> Jesus' life was about healing the whole person—body and spirit. . .

Church Health Center has cared for people in Memphis, we have seen that two-thirds of our patients seek treatment for illness that healthier living can prevent or control. We realized that if we want to make a lasting difference in our patients' lives, the most effective strategy is to encourage overall wellness in body and spirit. At a fundamental level, we must transform what the words *well* and *health* mean in the minds of most people.

To do that, we developed the Model for Healthy Living. Living healthy lives doesn't just mean that you see the doctor regularly. Rather, healthy living means that all aspects of your life are in balance. Your faith, work, nutrition, movement, family and friends, emotions, and medical health all contribute to a life filled with more joy, more love, and more connection with God.

How to Use This Book

This book provides opportunities to improve your health in whatever way you need to for your optimal wellness. For the next forty days, we invite you to be inspired by the real-life people whose lives have been changed by the Church Health Center. Each day offers us a new chance to improve our health, so each day we will give you helpful ways that you can make your life healthier.

Some days you may choose to focus on just one or two of our "tips": Faith Life, Medical, Movement, Work, Emotional, Family and Friends, or Nutrition. Some days you may want to try all of them. The important thing is to remember that God calls us to an abundant life, and we can always make changes to strive for our optimal wellness.

Forty days and numerous ways to live a healthy life—come and join us on the journey!

Eddie has been a fairly healthy individual. High

school football dominated his free time while he was growing up. As an adult, he continued to remain active through daily walks in his neighborhood and time at a local gym.

On Tuesday, June 6, 2006, Eddie was involved in a serious car accident. Six major operations and five months in the hospital left him confined to a wheelchair, and the possibility of amputation was very real. Many around him were not optimistic, but Eddie was hopeful that if he could get moving, he could save his legs and possibly run again.

Twelve months after the accident, Eddie came to Church Health Center in a wheelchair. For the next few months, Eddie committed his heart to the task of walking and eventually running. Through physical therapy and regular exercise, Eddie gradually built strength and flexibility in his legs. Eddie was regaining independence.

Over the next four months, Eddie was faithful to his recovery. He attended exercise sessions five days a week. He progressed from the bikes to standing to eventually walking for a few minutes on the treadmill. Excited by the results, he worked even harder to make progress.

Today Eddie continues his recovery. The physical effects of the accident only serve as a motivation to maintain his health. He walks at least five miles daily after his evening shift at work. At our Wellness Center, you are likely to find him on one of the treadmills, encouraging someone else to walk a few more steps.

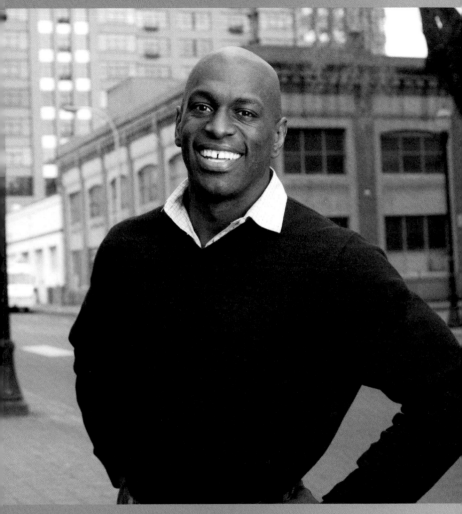

Many around him were not optimistic,
but Eddie was hopeful.

Morning Reflection

The beginning of a journey is always difficult. Change often happens slowly, and our minds and bodies may be reluctant to take the necessary steps to make positive change. Even the start of God's creation was somewhat chaotic—beginnings are not easy. But just as God created the world, He also created our bodies, and He will walk with us as we begin the journey toward wellness.

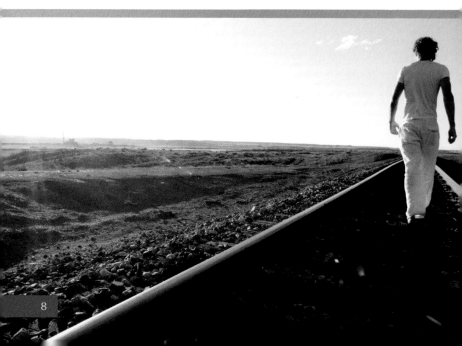

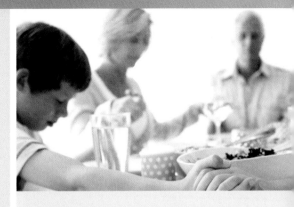

»Faith Life

Faith is an important part of overall wellness. Do you pray before meals? If you do not, start today. When we take a moment to return thanks to the One who has given us the food before we dig in, we acknowledge what we are putting into our bodies.

....

....

....

....

....

....

....

{ God walks with us as we begin the journey toward wellness. }

»Medical

Make a list of your medical concerns. If you have a history of high blood pressure, for example, write it down. This will help you to focus and set goals throughout the coming weeks.

1 ....

2 ....

3

»Movement

Go for a walk today. Do not exhaust yourself, and give yourself permission to stop when you feel you need to. Take note of where you stop so that you can note your progress as the journey progresses.

....

....

....

»Work

What is your work? It can be your job, volunteering, gardening, parenting, or any activity that gives meaning and structure to your days. Today, make a list of as many things as you can think of that make up your "work."

»Emotional

If you do not have a journal, take this opportunity to start one. You can use this book or a separate journal. But having a journal will give you the opportunity to sit and reflect on your experience on the journey to wellness.

»Family and Friends

Personal relationships, both family and friends, are crucial to overall wellness. They provide support, laughter, and engagement. Make a list of the personal relationships in your life on which you depend.

»Nutrition

What is your typical diet? Do you eat out a lot? Do you use a lot of prepared foods? Start a food journal or add "food journaling" to your current journal. This will help you as you set nutritional goals for yourself.

Evening Wrap-Up

Our bodies are created by God

and are a part of God's creation. And God called us "very good." God loves creation—all of creation—and so should we. But we often fall into the trap of not caring for ourselves as we should. As we set out on a journey to better health, we know that the way will not always be easy. We will certainly have moments of frustration as well as setbacks. But we can trust that God sees us as a part of creation and calls us "very good."

So God created mankin in his own image, in the image of God he created them; male and female he created them. . . . God saw all that he had made, and it was very good.

GENESIS 1:27, 31

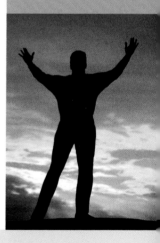

God of new beginnings, help me to see You in myself. As I begin this journey toward wellness, give me the wisdom to know that my body is Your creation. Thank You for this incredible gift, and help me to care for myself as You care for all of creation. In Your holy name, Amen.

Morning Reflection

When we set out on a trip, most often we get directions before we get in the car. But in order to get directions, we first need to know where we are starting. As we set out on this journey toward wellness, we need to know where we are now. Sometimes we start out on a good day, sometimes on a bad one. But whatever the day, we can know that God walks with us.

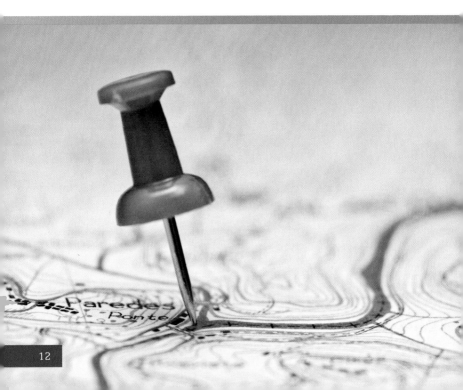

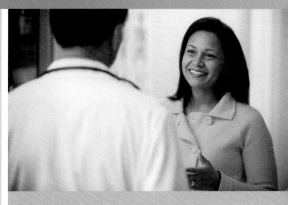

»Faith Life

What are ten words that you would use to describe your faith life right now? Take five minutes and write them down. Be honest, and be certain to include both the things that are positive about your faith life and a few things that are maybe less than positive.

....
....
....
....
....
....
....
....

> {
> As we set out on this journey toward wellness, we need to know where we are now.
> }

»Medical

When was your last physical by a medical doctor? If it has been over a year, call and make an appointment to get a checkup. It is important that you know your general state of health as you embark on this wellness journey.

....
....
....

»Movement

After your morning shower (so that your muscles are warm), do some light stretching. Bend over and see how close you can get to touching your toes. Where do your muscles feel tight? (Hint: Your stretching should feel comfortable. If any stretches hurt, pull back on the stretch.)

....
....

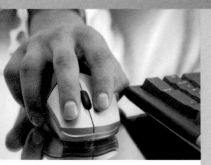

» Work

What do you like about your work? What do you dislike? Take five minutes and write some things that you like and dislike about the tasks you perform. (Remember, *work* is comprised of your job/career, but can also include volunteering, parenting, etc.)

» Emotional

Each day has a unique emotional makeup. Today, write in your journal about a time of the day when you experienced an emotional high and a time when you felt an emotional low. What were the events? What words would you use to describe them?

» Family and Friends

Do you eat family dinners? Family dinners are a wonderful way to spend time with your family, catching up and talking. They are also wonderful times to try new recipes. Take time today to plan a family dinner in the next week.

» Nutrition

Do you have a standard list for the grocery store? Make a list of things that you normally buy when you go to the store. In the days and weeks to come, change your grocery list based on the dietary suggestions in this book.

Evening Wrap-Up

Taking a close look at where we are can be a difficult task. Sometimes we may like what we see, and sometimes we may not. But the writer of Ecclesiastes tells us that when we like what we see, we should celebrate. And, when we perhaps do not like what we see, we should remember that God has made the world. God made every day—including the bad ones. What this means for us, even more than just that God has made the day, is that God has made our journey. God celebrates our successes and mourns our sorrows with us.

When times are good, be happy; but when times are bad, consider this: God has made the one as well as the other.

ECCLESIASTES 7:14

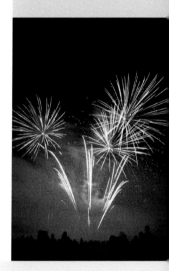

Dear Lord, thank You for the gift of all days, both good and bad. On this day, I pray that You would walk with me and give me direction as I set out on this journey toward wellness. In Your holy name, Amen.

Morning Reflection

Just as we must know where we are beginning when we set out on a journey, we also must have an idea of where we are going. On the journey toward wellness, it is important to have goals. Only with specific goals can we know what we are moving toward. Our goals may shift over time, but it is very important to know what our goals are.

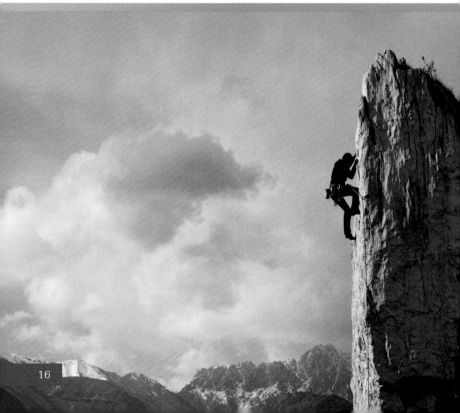

» Faith Life

How would you like to see your faith life change? Take five minutes today and write some changes that you would like to make in your faith life over the next six weeks.

» Medical

In light of the medical concerns you wrote down two days ago, how would you like to improve your medical health? For example, would you like to reduce the number of medications you are taking? Do you want to maintain your current state of health?

» Movement

Go for a walk today, and walk as far as you can walk. How much farther would you like to be able to walk in a week? In six weeks?

» Work

Return to the list you made yesterday of things you like and dislike about your work. What would you like to change about your work? What do you have the power and authority to change in your work?

» Emotional

If you start to feel overwhelmed today, sit down, close your eyes, and breathe deeply. Keep your breathing slow and even for a full minute. This will help your body to relax.

» Family and Friends

Are you embarking on this journey on your own or with a friend or some family members? Having a traveling companion can be very helpful. Think today about a friend or family member whom you might reach out to and invite to come along.

» Nutrition

What would you like to change about your nutritional habits? Eat less fat? Eat more vegetables? Maintain better portion control? Write down five nutritional goals for the next six weeks.

*Forgetting what
is behind and
straining toward
what is ahead,
I press on toward
the goal to win the
prize for which
God has called
me heavenward
in Christ Jesus.*

PHILIPPIANS
3:13–14

Evening Wrap-Up
We've all heard the phrase "eyes

on the prize." It is often used in a game or a race to encourage the players to focus on the end—the finish line—the prize. In Paul's letter to the Philippians, Paul is encouraging them to keep their eyes on the prize, "forgetting what is behind." While it is good to know where you have been and where you are beginning, there comes a point when we must let go of what is behind and look toward the outcome. On our journey toward wellness, it is time to let go of *what was*, and press on toward the goal of *what could be*.

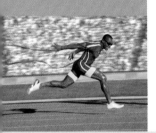

Loving God, give me focus today and all days. Help me to keep my eyes on the prize as I care for this wonderful body You have given me. In Your holy name, Amen.

Morning Reflection

We are still in the first days of this journey. But even four days in, the journey can begin to seem too much. Our expectations can (and do) shape our day-to-day experience of wellness and faith. Today we will spend some time considering what our expectations are of ourselves and of God as we continue on this journey toward wellness.

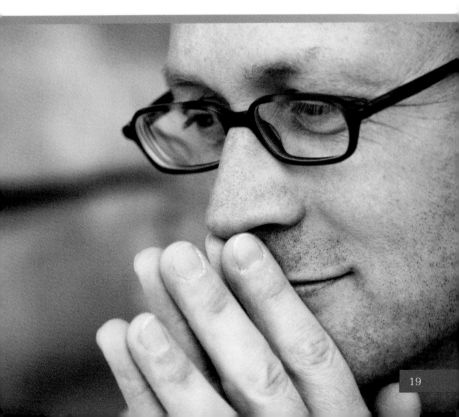

»Medical

If you do not know how to find your pulse, today is the day to learn! Use your index and middle fingers to feel your pulse at your wrist. Count the beats that you feel in fifteen seconds, and multiply the number by four. That is your standing heart rate.

....

....

....

....

»Movement

Spend ten minutes stretching today. Can you stretch a bit farther than you could a couple of days ago? What are your expectations for a couple of days from now?

....

....

....

»Faith Life

We all generally have expectations of God. Take five minutes and reflect honestly on the expectations that you have of God for this journey.

....

....

....

....

....

....

....

....

....

....

....

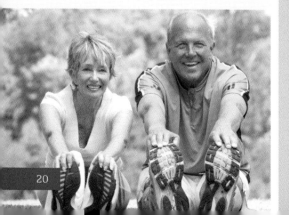

{ Today we will spend some time considering what our expectations are of ourselves and of God, }

»Work

What do you usually do on your breaks?
Do you drink coffee? Grab a snack from
the vending machine? Today go for a short
walk, or bring a healthy snack to work.

»Emotional

**Our expectations can seriously
impact our emotional well-being.** Take
five minutes and write in your journal about
what your expectations are for this journey
to wellness.

»Family and Friends

**Sometimes we can feel that our family
and friends have particular expectations
of us, and that can add to stress that we
are already feeling.** Today talk to a friend
or family member about your journey and
what your expectations are.

»Nutrition

What kind of food do you like to eat?
Take five minutes and make a list of your
favorite foods. Are they healthy foods?
Comfort foods? As this journey progresses,
you may be able to modify your favorite
foods to healthier versions.

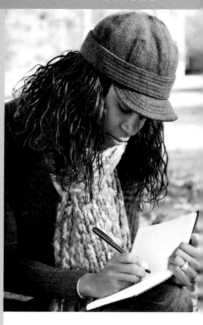

"Arise, shine, for your light has come, and the glory of the Lord rises upon you. See, darkness covers the earth and thick darkness is over the peoples, but the Lord rises upon you and his glory appears over you."

ISAIAH 60:1–2

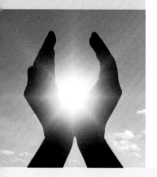

Evening Wrap-Up

We all have expectations of ourselves, both good and bad. But even our highest expectations are small compared to God's reality. God values each life, and if God so values us, we should surely value ourselves! Expectations are largely about realizing what we are capable of, and Isaiah reminds us that God's glory shines on us. With God's help, we are capable of anything. The journey to wellness may not always be an easy one, but it is certainly an achievable one.

Lord, on this journey to wellness, help me to have realistic expectations of myself and of You. But even more, help me always to see Your light that shines in me and in every darkness. In Your holy name, Amen.

Morning Reflection

Every journey begins with the first steps. To climb a mountain, we must begin at the base. We can never reach a summit without first starting at the bottom. Our journey toward wellness is all about taking steps—both literally and figuratively—toward better health. But in order to take those steps, we must decide on those first steps we will take.

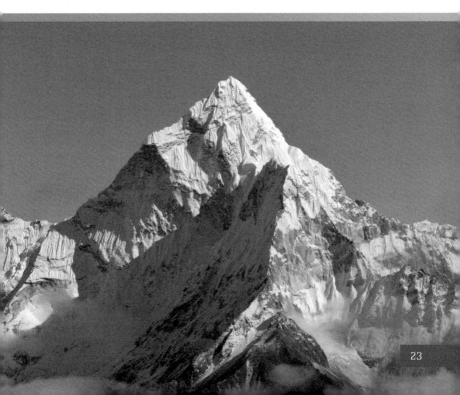

» Faith Life

Jesus knew a thing or two about taking first steps. Today, read the first chapter of the Gospel of Mark, the beginning of Jesus' earthly ministry. How does Jesus' beginning compare with the beginning of your journey toward wellness?

» Medical

Do you know what your blood pressure is? If you do not, make sure that you ask the next time you go to the doctor. Also, many drugstores have blood pressure machines if you would like to know sooner.

» Movement

Go for a walk today, a block or so farther than you did on Day 3. Again, do not exhaust yourself, but push your comfort limit a little.

» Work

Be certain to drink plenty of water throughout the day, even if you are really only sitting. When you stay hydrated, your body works better and you will have more energy and will feel better.

» Emotional

Taking first steps can be fairly intimidating. Do you feel fear? Excitement? Take five minutes today to sit and breathe, and focus on what you are feeling as you set out on this journey.

» Family and Friends

What kind of support do you need from your family and friends? Take a few minutes to identify the kind of support that would be most helpful from your personal relationships, and then talk to a friend or family member about it.

» Nutrition

One of the first steps toward good nutrition is to begin reading labels on the food that you buy and eat. Go to your pantry and read the labels on ten items, taking note of sodium content and the ingredient "high fructose corn syrup."

Evening Wrap-Up

Every project, each journey, begins with first steps. Even creation began with first steps. God had a starting point, a place where creation began. The first steps are sometimes tricky. And finding the motivation to take these steps when all we see in front of us is the steep incline of a mountain can be intimidating. But we can find comfort in the knowledge that God, too, has taken first steps. God can walk with us and give us strength on our first steps as we look up to the summit of the mountain.

In the beginning God created the heavens and the earth. Now the earth was formless and empty, darkness was over the surface of the deep, and the Spirit of God was hovering over the waters.

GENESIS 1:1–2

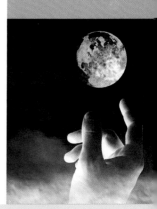

God of Strength, thank You for the gift of wellness. Help me to take the first steps toward health and wellness, and help me to remember that You walk with me in this beginning. In Your holy name, Amen.

Morning Reflection

We've all heard the phrase "two steps forward, one step back." It means that when we begin to make progress, it can feel like moving backward. Moving toward wellness can feel slow going, especially in the beginning. But we must trust that progress is being made and that, given enough time, we will begin to feel the difference.

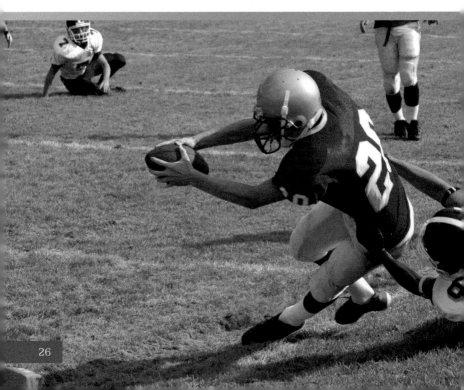

»Faith Life

Most of us have had both significant and minor setbacks in faith at some point in our lives. Think of a time when you experienced a setback in your faith life and how you managed to move forward.

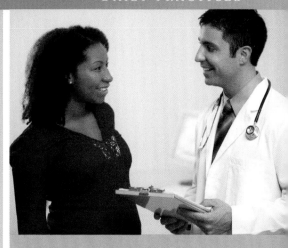

»Medical

While medical setbacks can be devastating, they need not be the end of the world. If you have had a medical setback, talk to your doctor about developing a strategy for moving forward.

»Movement

Spend ten minutes walking around your house (or walk around your neighborhood if you feel comfortable) taking two steps forward and one step backward. Notice that you still move forward. Also, walking backward exercises different muscles than walking forward.

{ Given enough time, we will begin to feel the difference. }

27

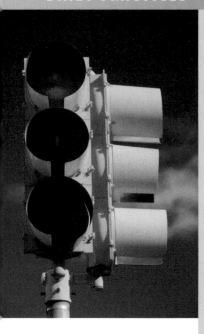

»Work

How do setbacks affect your work? Do you become less engaged in work? Or do you throw yourself into work? Using some kind of stress-relief tool (such as a stress ball or Silly Putty) can help you deal with setbacks at work.

»Emotional

Setbacks are perhaps the most devastating for our emotional health, because we can convince ourselves that moving forward from a setback is impossible. Today think of a strategy to deal with setbacks. (For example, decide to take a day off, go for a walk, and start again the next day.)

Family and Friends

» **Personal relationships are very important in the event of a setback, because they can offer you encouragement and perspective that you may not have for yourself.** Identify two people in your life who are particularly gifted in offering you encouragement when you need it.

Nutrition

» **Nutritional setbacks happen.** We give in to the temptation of a doughnut or eat too much out at a friend's birthday dinner. The temptation is to starve yourself the day after to "make up" for the setback. Instead, just get back on track eating a healthy and reasonable diet.

Evening Wrap-Up

Setbacks are a part of progress.

We live in a culture where results appear to be instantaneous. People undergo radical transformations in the span of a half hour television show. We often are not shown the waiting and the struggle moment by moment. Given this version of reality, it is no wonder that we consider every setback to be a failure! But Peter reminds us that God cares for us, and it is not for us to rise up on our own to overcome anxiety and obstacles. Instead, God will lift us up.

Humble yourselves, therefore, under God's mighty hand, that he may lift you up in due time. Cast all your anxiety on him because he cares for you.

1 PETER 5:6–7

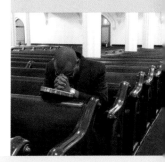

Merciful God, give me wisdom in the face of setbacks to realize that You lift me up. Help me to cast my anxiety on You as I continue on this journey to wellness. In Your holy name, Amen.

Morning Reflection

Congratulations! We have reached the end of the first week. We have taken the first steps toward wellness, and it is a week worthy of some celebration. As we celebrate, we can look forward to the rest of the journey and all of the adventures that we will have in the weeks to come.

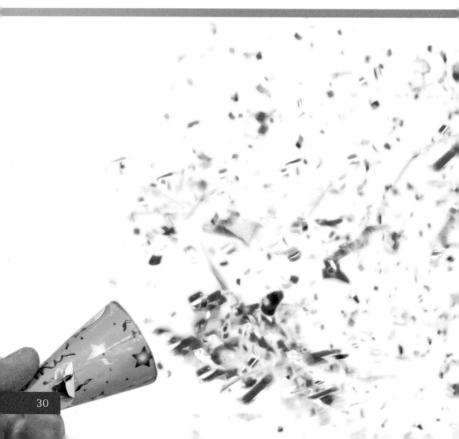

»Faith Life

Faith is an important part of wellness, but wellness is also important to faith. Keep in mind that God entered this world as a person with a body. Go for a walk today, and pray as you walk for God to be present in your body as well as your spirit.

....

....

....

....

....

....

....

....

{ Congratulations! We have reached the end of the first week. }

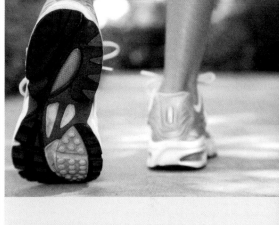

»Medical

Write down what your heart rate is when you have gone for a ten-minute walk around the block. Knowing this number will help as we move forward.

....

....

»Movement

Spend ten minutes in an activity that gets your heart rate up. Go for a walk, or do some jumping jacks. Try to make it an activity that you enjoy doing.

....

....

....

....

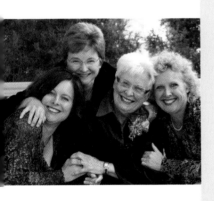

» Work

Take some small (two- or five-pound) hand weights to work to keep at your desk. If you have a minute or two, do a few sets of simple bicep curls to work your upper body a bit.

» Emotional

Write in your journal how you are feeling about the journey thus far. Are you excited? Tired? Encouraged? What does the "horizon" look like for you?

» Family and Friends

Have a small celebration with your family or some friends for getting through your first week. Do something that you enjoy doing with your family.

» Nutrition

Make a grocery list that looks forward. Include plenty of whole grains, fresh (or frozen) vegetables and fruits, and limit the prepared and processed foods. (Prepared and processed foods contain large amounts of sodium, sugar, and other additives.)

Evening Wrap-Up

This week, we have worked to define the "race set before us." We know the race, and we can predict at least a few of the obstacles along the way. But now it is time to run the race. As we run the race, God can give us perseverance and strength to travel the terrain, whatever we may encounter along the way. God can help us to let go of the things that hold us back so that we can turn our eyes to the horizon and enjoy the journey.

Therefore, since we are surrounded by such a great cloud of witnesses, let us throw off everything that hinders and the sin that so easily entangles. And let us run with perseverance the race marked out for us.

HEBREWS 12:1

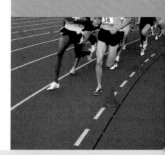

Lord God, *thank You for the gift of this body and the health that You have given me so far. Help me to run the race set before me.* In Jesus' name, Amen.

Frank was facing the facts about his weight and health honestly.

He was forty-five years old and weighed 358 pounds, and deep down he knew something had to change. The day of reckoning came when Frank said he got a "wake-up call" from his physician.

"He told me I needed to lose weight or else I was headed toward being a diabetic, having heart disease and hypertension. I wanted to do something about it," Frank said.

Since that day Frank has been putting one foot in front of the other—usually on a treadmill or elliptical exercise machine—six days a week. He also drinks water and eats lean meats (chicken and fish, baked or broiled) and lots of vegetables. A year later, his hard work has paid off. He's lost 127 pounds and is much healthier than he was a year ago.

The keys to Frank's success? "Prayer, determination, discipline, and dedication," he says. And as excited as Frank is about his success, he's just as excited about how God is using his success to inspire others.

"This blessing is not just for me," Frank said. "I want to be a blessing to someone else by encouraging them. That's why it doesn't bother me to take a minute when people stop me and ask, 'How did you do that?' Hey, we all need a little push, and that's what it's all about—building one another up."

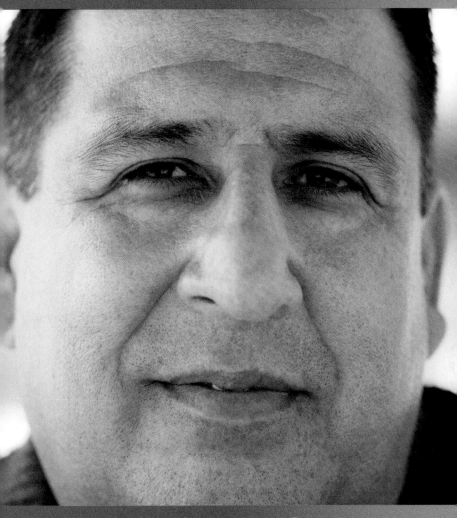

The keys to Frank's success?
"Prayer, determination, discipline,
and dedication."

Morning Reflection

Our state of wellness is very wrapped up in our habits—those behaviors that we engage in without even being totally aware of them. Today we will spend time reflecting on our habits and what we do on a day-to-day basis. Our habits can be so strongly ingrained that changing our behaviors can be very tricky. It involves focus, determination, and the occasional setback. Above all, we must know what our habits are, because when we know what our habits are, we can change them and better care for the bodies God has given us.

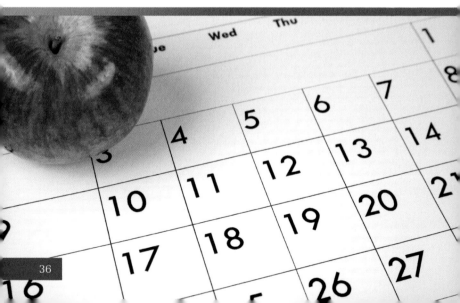

»Faith Life

Do you have a regular time when you pray?
Today, try praying at different times during the day. You may notice that you pray differently at different times of the day.

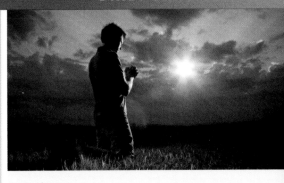

»Medical

Do you have a list of all your medications where it can be found? Make a list (either by hand or on a computer) and put it on your refrigerator. That way, if you ever have an emergency, your list of medications is readily available.

1
2
3

{ When we know what our habits are, we can change them. }

»Movement

When you go outside for a walk, do you wear sun block? Make sure when you spend time outside between the hours of 10:00 a.m. and 4:00 p.m. that you protect yourself from the sun, especially your nose, ears, and cheeks.

»Work

What are your habits when you get home from work? Do you eat? Clean? Watch television? Pay attention today to the small things that you do. Write down your actions in fifteen-minute increments. You may be surprised!

»Emotional

We often have emotional ups and downs over the course of the day. Today, pay special attention to when you feel those highs and lows. How do you feel in the morning? After lunch? In the evening? Write down in your journal when you have your highs and lows.

»Family and Friends

Do you have things that you often do with your family and friends? What are they? Spend a few minutes and write a list of the things that you like to do with the people in your life.

»Nutrition

Don't drink your calories! Substitute water for sweetened drinks such as sweetened iced tea or soda. If you want something fizzy, try drinking seltzer water instead of plain water.

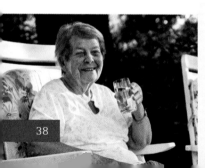

Evening Wrap-Up

We can change bad habits, and we can establish good ones. In his letter to the Colossians, Paul encourages us to lay down our bad habits in favor of good habits. He urges us to lay down our old selves—the selves of the bad habits—and clothe ourselves in the new self. As we continue on this journey toward wellness, we can look to this encouragement from Paul to change our habits. We can strive toward recognizing those behaviors that we must "lay down" and toward clothing ourselves with better habits.

As God's chosen ones, holy and beloved, clothe yourselves with compassion, kindness, humility, meekness, and patience. Bear with one another and, if anyone has a complaint against another, forgive each other. . . . Above all, clothe yourselves with love, which binds everything together in perfect harmony.

COLOSSIANS 3:12–14 NRSV

God of Patience, help me today to be patient with myself as I lay down my old habits in favor of better ones. Help me to better care for my body, recognizing that it is a gift from You. In Your holy name, Amen.

Morning Reflection

Yesterday we explored what our habits are. But in addition to our habits, we need to address our triggers. Triggers are emotions or events that "turn on" our habits. Some triggers can be stress, sadness, boredom, and even happiness. Like our habits, triggers are so deeply ingrained that they can be almost invisible. So once again, the key to changing behavioral triggers is to know what they are. Today we will focus on those behavioral triggers and on what we can do to change them.

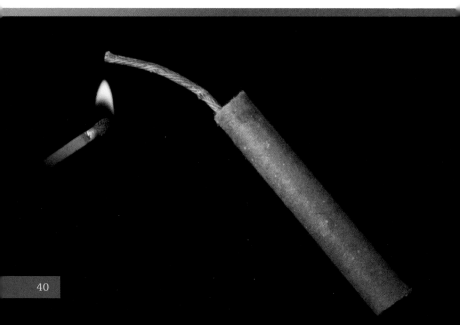

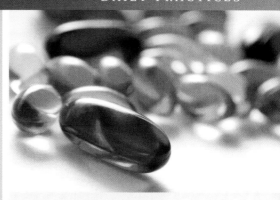

»Faith Life

Often as a part of our faith life, we neglect to sit quietly and listen or meditate. Today spend five minutes sitting quietly and breathing. Try to quiet your inner voice and just listen.

....
....
....
....
....
....
....
....
....

»Medical

In addition to having a list of your medications posted on your refrigerator, make sure that a close relative or friend has a list of your medications and recommended dosages.

....
....
....

»Movement

Many of us eat when we feel bored or overwhelmed. Today if you feel bored (but are not actually hungry), instead of snacking, try doing some simple stretches such as rolling your neck or stretching your arms.

....
....
....
....

{ Triggers are emotions or events that "turn on" our habits. }

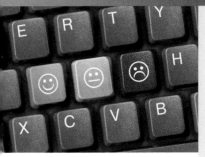

» Work

What are your triggers at work? Do you always take a coffee break at a certain time? Eat a lunch from a vending machine? Try replacing your coffee break with herbal tea, and bring a lunch from home.

» Emotional

What do you do when you feel happy? When you feel sad? When you are bored? Take five minutes and write in your journal, thinking about how you usually behave when faced with these emotions.

» Family and Friends

Family can be one of the biggest triggers of all, because when families get together, we have long-standing patterns of behavior, emotion—and especially eating! Today, if your family is gathering, try to focus on the fellowship rather than on food.

» Nutrition

If you do feel like snacking today, try snacking on some unsalted nuts or dried fruits instead of sugary or salty snacks like cookies and chips. Make sure you enjoy the proper serving size.

Evening Wrap-Up

When faced with our triggers, we may feel out of control. These behaviors can take over even when we do not seem to be making a conscious decision! We might blame our habits and triggers when we are at our weakest. But the psalmist has a word of assurance for us: "You rescue the poor from those too strong for them." God gives us strength when we are weakest. So as we identify our triggers, it can only be to our advantage to lean on God in times of weakness.

Then my soul will rejoice in the LORD and delight in his salvation. My whole being will exclaim, "Who is like you, LORD? You rescue the poor from those too strong for them, the poor and needy from those who rob them."

PSALM 35:9–10

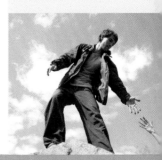

Lord God, help me to lean on You for the strength and wisdom I need as I challenge my habits and trigger behaviors. In Your holy name, Amen.

Morning Reflection

A cluttered desk is evidence of a cluttered mind,

at least according to this small piece of common wisdom. When our minds are full of chatter—worry, confusion, stress—we lack focus. When our lives (and kitchens!) are full of clutter, we can have a difficult time focusing on the importance of wellness. Today we will focus on cleaning house, both literally and figuratively in all aspects of wellness. As we clear away the clutter, we make room for the things that are healthy and make our lives more wellness oriented.

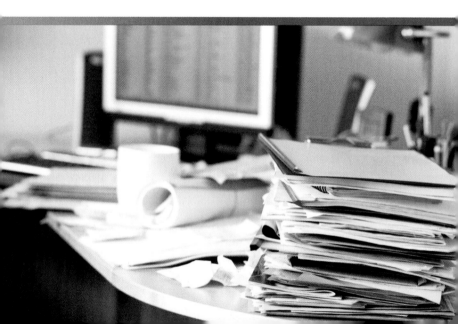

» Faith Life

Yesterday you spent time meditating and listening. Today, spend ten minutes sitting quietly again. Try to quiet your mind, clear out the clutter—the stress and anxiety. Breathe and let God in.

» Medical

When was the last time you cleaned out your medicine cabinet? Lots of accidents can be avoided by disposing of expired and old medication. Today take inventory of your medicine cabinet and throw out anything expired or unusable.

» Movement

Is a messy house or room keeping you from exercising or eating properly? Spend a half hour today decluttering one area of your house. When you are finished, you might feel better and less overwhelmed.

» Work

Clear out a space at your work (in your desk or somewhere convenient) where you can keep some healthy snacks on hand. When you take a break, instead of going to a vending machine, enjoy a healthy snack and a short walk.

» Emotional

Set aside some time today to take a warm bath. Even spending a few minutes soaking in a bath can help to relax your muscles. Do some deep breathing as you soak.

» Family and Friends

Recruit some of your family and friends to help you clean out your kitchen. Throw out expired foods, as well as processed foods with high sugar or fat content.

» Nutrition

Move the unhealthy snacks, such as potato chips or cookies, out of reach. Set them on a high shelf in the pantry or throw them out entirely. Move healthy snacks, such as fresh vegetables or fruits, into easy-to-grab places.

Evening Wrap-Up

As we progress on this journey,

there will be times when we will have to stop and—literally or figuratively—clean house. After all, life happens and things pile up. But if we do not take a day (or even one hour) now and then to clear the decks, we will become overwhelmed and our progress will come to a standstill. Remember that we are most likely to fall back into old habits because they're what we know best. But Proverbs reminds us that before we build a house, we need first to do our planning and preparation. In the journey to wellness, that means clearing space in our minds, hearts, and homes for wellness to be a priority.

Put your outdoor work in order and get your fields ready; after that, build your house.

PROVERBS 24:27

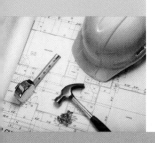

God of Balance, help me to prepare my heart, mind, and home for a wellness-oriented life. Help me to clean out the clutter so that I can build a strong foundation for wellness. In Your holy name, Amen.

Morning Reflection

Our overall wellness is dependent on our _attitude_ toward wellness. If our attitude is defeatist, then forward motion will be very difficult. However, if we approach wellness with confidence, we are more likely to be consistent, to roll with setbacks as they come, and to understand wellness in its entirety, rather than as individual parts. The journey to wellness is not always easy, but with a positive attitude, the path might smooth out on those days when we are having a particularly difficult time.

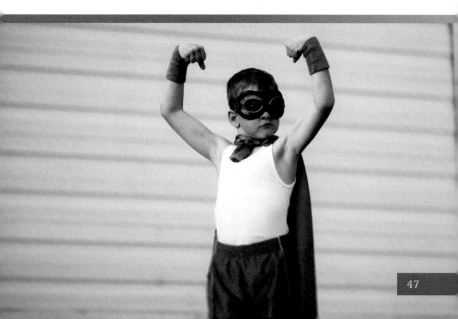

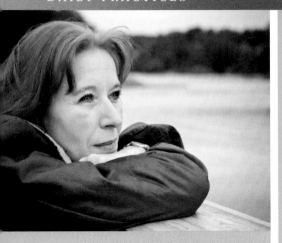

»Faith Life

Take five minutes today and meditate again. Quiet your thoughts, and then focus on the blessings that you have received, such as a body that works, wonderful friends, good food.

»Medical

Remember that medications can have side effects—some are physical and some are emotional. If you are having emotional side effects (such as depression, anxiety, hyperactivity) or physical side effects, let your doctor know as soon as possible.

»Movement

Exercise can lift your mood. If you are feeling negative, try doing thirty jumping jacks, and then stretch your arms and your back. Even a small amount of exercise can help you to feel more awake and more positive.

Our overall wellness is dependent on our attitude toward wellness.

»Work

Having a difficult day at work? Instead of focusing on the negative, think of something fun that you can do when you get home, even if it is simply getting outside to enjoy the fresh air. Write it down in a place where you can see your plans for your evening.

»Emotional

Sleep deprivation can get in the way of having a good attitude. When we are tired, our bodies and brains do not function well. Try to get a good night's sleep, even if it means leaving something undone in your day. You'll feel better when you wake up!

»Family and Friends

Friends are a wonderful resource for dealing with negativity. If you are feeling stressed or overwhelmed, try calling a friend for an emotional pick-me-up. Better yet, suggest that you go for a walk with your friend.

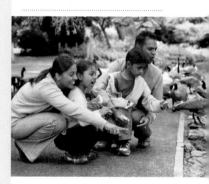

»Nutrition

Cook yourself a delicious and healthy meal, such as whole-grain pasta or lean meat with steamed vegetables. Eating well helps us feel better and can help us keep a positive attitude.

> "By the tender mercy of our God, the dawn from on high will break upon us, to give light to those who sit in darkness and in the shadow of death, to guide our feet into the way of peace."
>
> LUKE 1:78–79
> NRSV

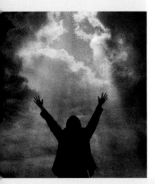

Evening Wrap-Up

God walks with us on this road to wellness.

In this passage from the Gospel of Luke, we know that God's light will shine on those who sit in darkness. It is not always easy, and it is certainly not automatic, to get up in the morning with a positive attitude. And some days will be better than others. But if we can remember every day that God shines in the darkness, then we may find encouragement in God's light even if we can't muster up the positive attitude for ourselves.

God of light, help me to see Your light in the darkness. Give me a positive attitude as I walk on this journey toward wellness. In Your holy name, Amen.

Morning Reflection

Wellness is about wholeness. It is about taking care of your whole person. When we only care for some parts of ourselves and neglect other parts, we do not care for the whole self. But God created us as whole selves—body and spirit—and so we ought to care for the entire self as well. Today we will focus on ways to appreciate and care for the entire self rather than individual, separate parts.

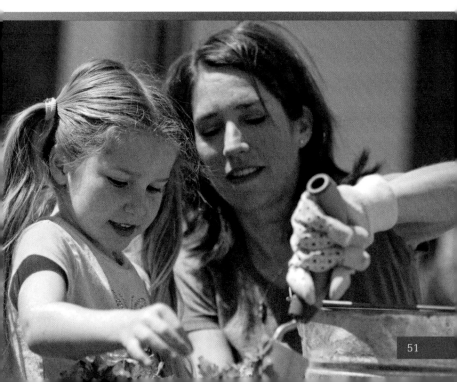

» Faith Life

When you pray today, wiggle your fingers and your toes. Stand up and sit down. Jump up and down. Breathe in and out. Think about how our whole bodies can pray, rather than just our minds or our spirits.

» Medical

In addition to prescription medication, do you take over-the-counter medication and/or vitamins? Include those on your list of medications for the refrigerator and emergency contact. Tell your doctor about those, too.

» Movement

Put on some music. Spend five minutes today dancing to the music in whatever way you can dance. Move your whole body as much as you can. Move your head, your back, your fingers, your toes. Feel your entire body working together.

» Work

Most of us work using one aspect of our personality more than other parts. Today, try to take five minutes at work and use another aspect of your body or personality. If you sit at a computer all day, go for a short walk. If you're on the phone, take a moment to stretch, and if you stand all day, find a quiet place to sit.

» Emotional

Sometimes, we can feel pulled in seventeen different directions at the same time. To pull yourself together and feel whole, take a shower and let yourself relax and breathe before getting back to your life.

» Family and Friends

Healthy relationships are very important to wellness and to wholeness. Today spend some time enjoying the company of your family and friends. Forget about the "shoulds"—just enjoy socializing and having fun!

» Nutrition

Just as there are many parts to a person, balanced nutrition includes nutrients from a variety of foods. Make sure when you prepare meals that you include fruits and vegetables, lean protein, and whole-grain carbohydrates.

Evening Wrap-Up

God created us whole. In his letter to the Corinthians, Paul reminds us of how God designed our bodies. No part of the body, he writes, is necessarily better than any other part of the body. Instead, each part of the body is a part for the whole—and it is the whole that we are concerned with today. As we move forward on this journey, we must keep in mind that God creates us as whole beings—body and spirit. It is our role to care for God's creation, including our whole body.

If the whole body were an eye, where would the sense of hearing be? If the whole body were an ear, where would the sense of smell be? But in fact God has placed the parts in the body, every one of them, just as he wanted them to be.

1 CORINTHIANS 12:17–18

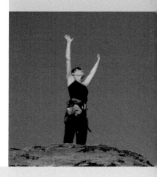

God of wholeness, thank You for the wonderful gift of my body and for Your wisdom that was used in creating me. Help me today to see myself as You do. In Your holy name, Amen.

Morning Reflection

Often when we think about wellness, we focus on what will be difficult on the journey—losing weight, exercising, depriving ourselves of foods we love. But while the journey does have its difficulties, we need not focus solely on the hard parts. So today we will turn our focus to the enjoyment that we can experience as a part of the journey to wellness. Wellness is not merely about deprivation. It is about being able to fully enjoy the life that we have been given.

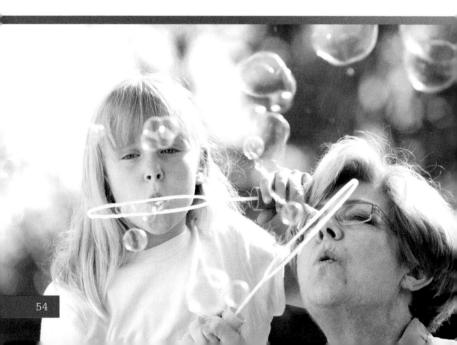

»Faith Life

Prayer and meditation do not always have to be somber and solemn. Laughter and fun and rejoicing need to be a part of our faith life. Think of something funny that has happened, and thank God for giving us humor in our lives.

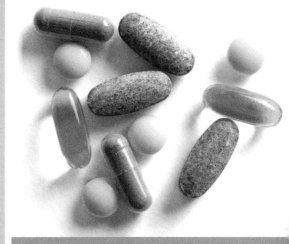

»Medical

Some vitamins and supplements can keep us healthy rather than trying to fix what is wrong. Ask your doctor about some vitamin supplements that can potentially improve your health.

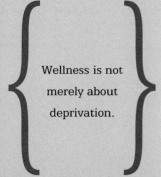

Wellness is not merely about deprivation.

»Movement

Spend some time today doing something you enjoy. Go for a walk or dance around your house. Having fun while exercising makes it more likely that you will continue exercising.

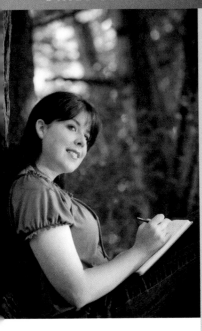

» Work

We do not often think of work as something to enjoy. Today find something that you enjoy about being at work, and focus on that. If you cannot think of something, try going for a walk or stepping outside when you have a break.

» Emotional

When we do not take the time to enjoy ourselves, we can become overwhelmed. Today spend five minutes writing in your journal about the things that you enjoy doing.

» Family and Friends

Tonight enjoy an evening out with your family or friends. Go to a healthy restaurant, and try something on the menu that you may not have had otherwise.

» Nutrition

Instead of potato chips and a cream-based dip (like onion dip), try making salsa and eating it with baked tortilla chips for a delicious and healthy party snack.

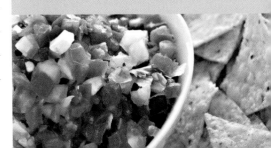

Evening Wrap-Up

Just as a difficult path can be part of the journey toward wellness, so

can enjoyment. If we enjoy ourselves, we are more likely to move toward wellness and less likely to resent wellness in our lives. After all, wellness is often about feeling good. God wants enjoyment and rejoicing for us. In fact, we have been created for rejoicing! Paul tells us in his letter to the Romans to be ardent in spirit and to rejoice in hope. As we spend our energy rejoicing and enjoying the path to wellness, we will feel better about ourselves and with God.

Never be lacking in zeal, but keep your spiritual fervor, serving the Lord. Be joyful in hope, patient in affliction, faithful in prayer.

ROMANS 12:11–12

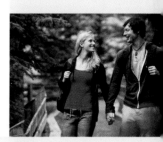

Living God, thank You for this journey and for helping me through my tough days so far. Help me now to see You in this journey and to enjoy this path. In Your holy name, Amen.

Morning Reflection

At the end of another week, today we can pause and give thanks for the gifts that God has given us: wonderful food, family and friends, bodies that move and work. When we stop to give thanks, it feels good. And when we give thanks, we have to stop for a moment, take stock, and appreciate what we have. This can give us motivation to move forward on our journey toward the next thing. So today, we give thanks for the week past and look forward to the weeks to come.

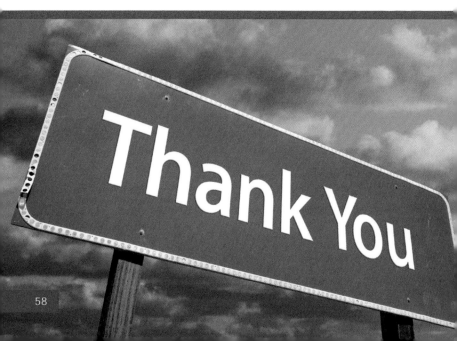

»Faith Life

Thankfulness comes in a variety of forms. Today make a list of everything that you encounter for which you are thankful. At the end of the day, say a prayer, reading the list.

When we stop
to give thanks,
it feels good.

»Medical

Refilling prescriptions can be difficult to remember. If your pharmacy has an automatic refill program, take advantage of it. This way, you are less likely to run out of your medication.

»Movement

If you are waiting in line today, spend time in line rising up on your toes and lowering back down. This helps to strengthen your calf muscles, which will help build walking endurance.

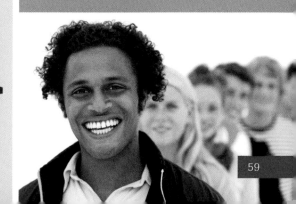

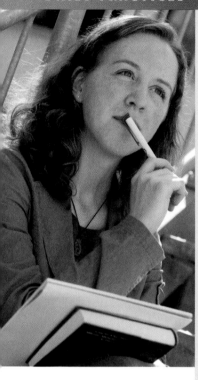

»Work

As you work today, spend some time thinking about the things for which you are thankful. Go for a walk when you are on a break and give thanks for the time you spend walking.

»Emotional

When you are feeling overwhelmed or upset, spend five minutes remembering and making a list of the things for which you are thankful. This can help you gain perspective.

»Family and Friends

Today take a moment to thank your family and friends for the support they give you. Remember that they are a very important part of your overall wellness.

»Nutrition

If you are a soda drinker and find it difficult to give up the habit, try drinking seltzer water for a carbonated treat. If you want something sweet, try adding a small amount of no-sugar-added fruit juice to the seltzer.

Evening Wrap-Up

The Lord is good, and for this, we give thanks! We can give thanks for each day, for the meals on our table, for the family and friends who love us. We can certainly give thanks for all of God's blessings. Giving thanks and being thankful on the journey toward wellness, we are bound to get overwhelmed. Wellness means changing habits and sometimes giving up things that we have always done and enjoyed. Giving thanks helps us to take stock of what we have been given. If we take the time to give thanks, we may find ourselves more grateful.

"Give thanks to the LORD Almighty, for the LORD is good; his love endures forever."

JEREMIAH 33:11

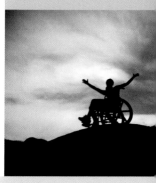

Life-giving God, please make me thankful today. Help me to take the time to be grateful. Help me to see all of the blessings in my life. In Your holy name, Amen.

Iva weighed 437 pounds. She had diabetes that re-

quired her to take up to 140 units of insulin a day. Iva knew that she needed to lose weight. So she started skipping meals and starving herself. She then became depressed, even suicidal, and knew there had to be a better way.

When she sought help, she began eating—with a focus on wellness—and started losing weight. Iva's thirty-year-old daughter, Ella, noticed a difference when Iva became pickier at the grocery store. "She started reading food labels and saying, 'This has too much sodium,' " Ella said. "She brought home all sorts of herbs and spices from the store and great recipes. . .and was just cooking away. Her spirit was totally different."

Now, with a new wellness-oriented diet and exercise plan, Iva has lost over 200 pounds, and she is still losing weight! Just as important, she manages her diabetes with only oral medica-tion, and her body is processing sugars better than a person without diabetes. Asked about how her new, healthy lifestyle has changed her life, Iva says, "When my pastor sees me now, he just smiles and says, 'Iva, God is good,' and I say, 'Tell me about it.' I am living a life I had only dreamed of."

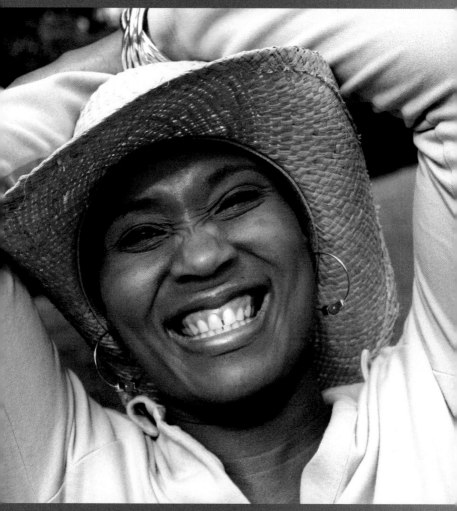

"I say, 'Tell me about it.' I am living a life I had only dreamed of."

Morning Reflection

Wellness is about balance—something that Iva learned firsthand. By not eating, Iva lost weight, but she was not getting healthier. She had to find the balance that worked for her life. We also have to find the balance in our own lives, with our bodies, with God. After all, Ecclesiastes tells us that there is a time for every purpose under heaven. What an encouragement to seek balance in the lives God has given us!

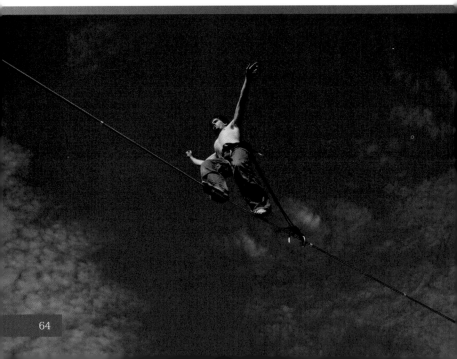

»Faith Life

Read Ecclesiastes 3:1 and take a walk, noticing the careful balance of God's creation. What do you see? What do you hear? What do you smell? Where do you think you fit in the balance?

....

....

....

....

....

....

....

....

....

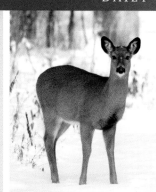

»Medical

Your physical health is about achieving a balance between medications and lifestyle—between your doctor and you. Today write some questions that you can ask your doctor the next time you go in for a checkup.

....

....

....

{ There is a time for every purpose under heaven. }

»Movement

There is no movement without balance! Spend a few minutes today exercising your balance by standing on one leg (three minutes on one and then three on the other). Use a chair or countertop for support if you need it.

....

....

»Work

Balancing work and wellness can be difficult. Today try to add some "wellness balance" to your workday. Take a couple of short walks around the office, or even just take a couple of moments in the day to breathe and relax.

»Emotional

Emotional balance is sometimes very difficult to maintain, especially with a busy schedule. Today find five minutes to balance your business with some quiet time. Spend five minutes sitting and relaxing. Take some deep breaths in and out, close your eyes, and relax.

»Family and Friends

Finding and maintaining your balance is at least partially about knowing when you need to reach out for support. Today try to go for a brisk walk with a friend or a member of your family.

»Nutrition

We've all heard of a well-balanced diet. Good nutrition is mostly about balance, and balance is about moderation. Portion size can make a huge difference in whether you gain, lose, or maintain weight. Today keep a log of the things you eat, paying attention to portion size.

Evening Wrap-Up

Finding balance in life is tough,

but it is important nonetheless. At those times when you are feeling completely out of balance (which happens even to the most centered and balanced people from time to time), remember that God keeps all of creation in balance. Because of that, you can trust that you are cared for even when you feel out of control.

Who has measured the waters in the hollow of his hand, or with the breadth of his hand marked off the heavens? Who has held the dust of the earth in a basket, or weighed the mountains on the scales and the hills in a balance?

ISAIAH 40:12

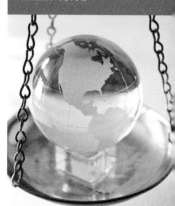

Lord, help me to find balance in all the many facets of my life. Make me aware of the balance of Your creation and the care that You show for me in that balance. Help me to live a healthier and more balanced life, caring for myself the way You care for all of creation. Amen.

Morning Reflection

Balance is an attempt to walk the middle path. Keep in mind, Iva began her weight-loss journey by starving herself. She actually became healthier when she decided to eat more often! So, *balance* is not about extremes, but about moderation. In wellness the temptation is to think that we must "be strong" and "do it alone." But Jesus has assured us that "with God, all things are possible." God's grace is such that we never need to "go it alone." Thus, God gives us a graceful balance of vulnerability, strength, and support.

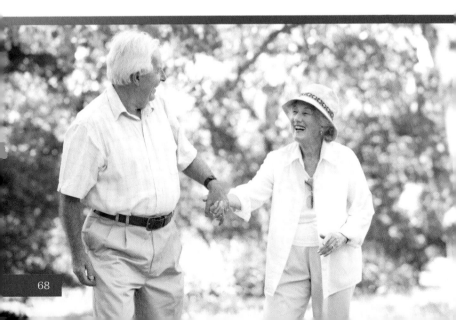

»Faith Life

Discouragement and setbacks are a part of life. Read Matthew 19:26. Do any of your goals feel impossible? Have you experienced setbacks? Go for a walk and try to grant yourself some grace as God grants grace to all of us.

....

....

....

....

....

....

....

....

{

Balance is not about extremes, but about moderation.

}

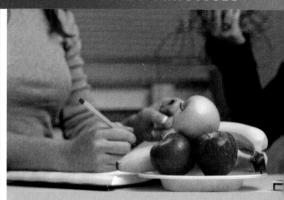

»Medical

Our medical model is often based on what we must do. Exercise, eat right, and take the right medications. But just as important is rest. Sleep gives your body the energy to function properly. Today try to give yourself some rest.

....

....

....

»Movement

Not all exercise has to involve sweating! Today continue to work on your balance by spending ten minutes stretching. Try to touch your toes, get on the floor and stretch your back by pushing up on your arms, and reach each of your arms across your chest.

....

....

....

» Work

Do you work in an office where someone is always bringing in treats? Birthday cake, donuts, and bagels can be trouble. Balance out these unhealthy snacks by bringing in a fruit plate to share. Maybe you'll inspire others to bring in healthier snacks next time!

» Emotional

When we're trying to get into new habits, it is easy to become overwhelmed and, in turn, to fall back on old, comfortable habits. Take a slow walk today, focusing on your breathing, and let go of the things that leave you overwhelmed.

» Family and Friends

Family dinners are a wonderful place to begin wellness-oriented and balanced meals. Today, plan a family dinner that contains mostly vegetables, a reasonable serving size of protein (like a lean meat), and a small serving of whole grains (rice, barley, whole-wheat pasta).

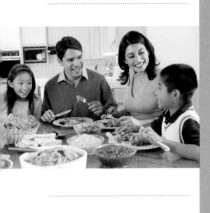

» Nutrition

Depriving yourself entirely of the foods you love is more likely to push you to binge. Balance strict food intake and calorie counting with an occasional small treat. Today, treat yourself to a sensible treat, such as a scoop of low-fat frozen yogurt or a cup of raspberries.

Evening Wrap-Up

Paul reminds us of the balance that exists in strength and weakness. This reminder is good to consider any time you try to form a new habit. Admitting your own powerlessness gives strength beyond what you might know you have. God's strength is present in your weakness. Therefore, do not fight your weaknesses. Setbacks and discouragement may feel impossible, but with God, "all things are possible."

"My grace is sufficient for you, for my power is made perfect in weakness." Therefore I will boast all the more gladly about my weaknesses, so that Christ's power may rest on me. That is why, for Christ's sake, I delight in weaknesses. . . . For when I am weak, then I am strong.

2 CORINTHIANS 12:9–10

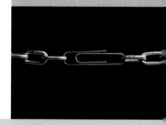

Lord, help me to recognize the possibilities that Your grace provides for me. When I feel discouraged or when I have setbacks, help me to balance my own disappointments with the same grace that You show me and all my brothers and sisters. Amen.

Morning Reflection

When we think about wellness, we often think only about numbers on a scale. And certainly, weight is a part of an overall wellness-oriented lifestyle. However, wellness is really about balancing all aspects of your person. In particular, wellness is about incorporating all senses. After all, God has blessed us with the senses of sight, smell, sound, taste, and touch. It makes sense, then, that a wellness-oriented lifestyle includes all of our senses—not just a number on the scale.

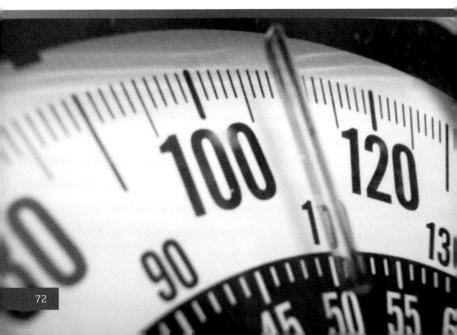

» Faith Life

Psalm 34:8 reads, "Taste and see that the LORD is good; blessed is the one who takes refuge in him." Today say a prayer before every meal. Remember that God cares about every aspect of our lives, including our food.

» Medical

Before changing her life, Iva had to identify her medical issues. Today ask yourself how you feel in general so that you can discuss it with your doctor. Are you energetic or tired? Do you feel good moving around, or do you often feel short of breath?

» Movement

Today try to embrace all of your senses as you go for a walk around your neighborhood. Observe all of the colors, smells, and even tastes as you walk. But mostly, feel the air on your skin and feel the movement in your body.

» Work

We often focus on the negative effects of work, but working—being active and positively engaged—is an important component of wellness. Today try to focus on the positive engagement in your work—whether you work in an office or at home.

» Emotional

Emotions always have a significant effect on wellness, both for better and for worse. Sometimes emotions can get out of control and we can lose perspective on the big picture. Today go for a walk and reflect on your "big picture." What is important to you? What is not?

» Family and Friends

Healthy relationships can bring balance to your life in many ways, but especially by offering fellowship and fun. Today call a friend or a family member and have some fun by dancing to some music or shopping at a farmers' market for some fresh local produce.

» Nutrition

Healthy food, especially when you use fresh ingredients and healthy spices, does not need to taste bad. Today make a meal using fresh vegetables, healthy fats, and lean proteins. Don't forget to season it with some fresh herbs!

Then God said, "I give you every seed-bearing plant on the face of the whole earth and every tree that has fruit with seed in it. They will be yours for food. And to all the beasts of the earth and all the birds in the sky and all the creatures that move along the ground—everything that has the breath of life in it—I give every green plant for food." And it was so.

GENESIS 1:29–30

Evening Wrap-Up

God has filled this world with beauty in sight, sound, fragrance, taste, and touch. It is no wonder that all of our senses are involved in wellness—God created us that way! When we live wellness-oriented lives, we live lives balanced in all of God's creation.

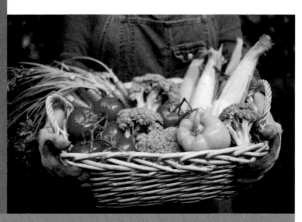

Lord God, You have filled my life with beautiful colors and delicious tastes and smells. Help me to live my life in the fullness of Your creation by taking the time to notice the wonder You have created around me. Amen.

Morning Reflection

To begin living a wellness-oriented life, Iva had to reach outside her comfort zone. She had to try foods she had never tried before. She had to exercise. She even had to relate differently to her friends and family. Wellness is about changing an entire lifestyle, which means that we must venture beyond the things we are accustomed to. Today we will focus on moving beyond our comfort zone and into the wellness zone.

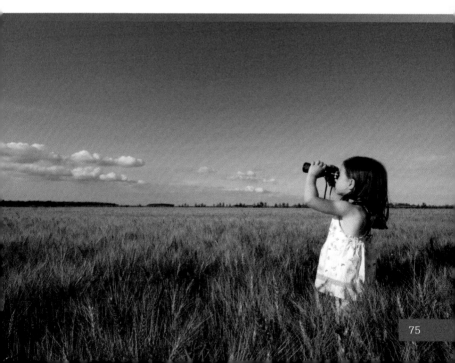

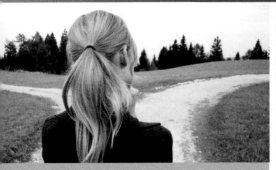

»Medical

Do you know the symptoms of stroke?
They include weakness in an arm, hand, or
leg; loss of feeling on one side of the body;
blindness in one eye; difficulty talking; loss of
balance. Familiarize yourself with the symptoms of major illnesses or events so that you
can recognize them in your own health or in
the health of those around you.

»Movement

**A healthy exercise regimen consists of
building our aerobic strength, muscular
strength and endurance, and flexibility.**
Today, do three sets of ten wall push-ups to
start building your upper-body strength.

»Faith Life

**Have you ever felt called
to leave your comfort
zone?** How did you handle
it? Do you feel that God
walked with you? Spend five
minutes today meditating on
how God has acted in your
life outside your comfort
zone.

{
Wellness is about
changing an
entire lifestyle.
}

»Work

Good posture helps you to breathe, increases strength in your back and abdomen, and can help decrease back pain and headaches. Today at work, try to remind yourself to keep your head up and your shoulders back and relaxed.

»Emotional

Leaving the comfort zone is a hugely emotional experience. It can cause a great deal of anxiety or even panic. If you feel anxious about leaving your comfort zone, slow down, take a deep breath, and remember that you are safe.

»Family and Friends

Leaving your comfort zone can be less intimidating if you have family and friends to do it with you. Today go for a walk with a friend or family member. Try to walk farther and at a brisker pace than you usually do.

»Nutrition

Eating a wellness-oriented diet can mean leaving behind food habits that have been comfortable for a long time. Today be particularly mindful of portion size as you eat. For example, a serving of meat should only be about the size of a deck of cards.

Evening Wrap-Up

"When my life was ebbing away, I remembered you, LORD, and my prayer rose to you, to your holy temple."

JONAH 2:7

Last week we explored habits, so we know just how powerful those habits can be. But even more than just powerful, our habits are comfortable, which makes it difficult to try something new. Yet there are times in our lives when we are called to leave our comfort zones. Consider Jonah, who ran away when God asked him to go to Nineveh. Now, while most of us will not be swallowed by a giant fish, getting out to exercise can feel like just as tall an order as going to Nineveh! However, in order to grow, we must stretch and extend ourselves into unknown territories, knowing all the while that God walks with us.

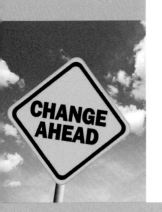

God of new journeys, thank You for being a God who calls me into unfamiliar places. Help me today to step outside my comfort zone and embrace change in my life. In Your holy name, Amen.

Morning Reflection

As we continue on the journey toward wellness, we need to take some time, occasionally, to revisit the goals that we set in the first week. That is, we need to remember our purpose for being on this journey. Is it to lose weight? To reduce the number of medications we're on? To feel better all around? (Remember, purposes will be different from person to person and perhaps even from day to day.) So today we will work on touching base once again with our purpose on the journey.

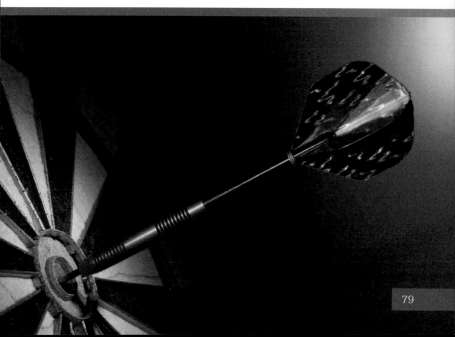

» Faith Life

Do you remember what your goals were for your faith life in week one? Today go back and read your goals, and then write for five minutes about your progress. Are your goals still the same? Have they changed?

» Medical

Do you know your family history? If your parents, grandparents, aunts, or uncles have or had an illness, it can be relevant to your own health. Heart disease, diabetes, and cancers are particularly important to know.

» Movement

We all like to relax by watching television or reading a book. Today while you watch television, try doing some bicep curls with hand weights, or do several sets of squats.

» Work

Take a copy of that list of prescription drugs, vitamins, over-the-counter medications, and family history to keep at work. Also, if possible, have a place at work where you can keep the medication that you need during the day, instead of taking your medication with you to work and back home every day.

» Emotional

Going through periods of change can be particularly taxing on our emotions. Connecting with our purpose can help us gain some stability. Today spend ten minutes writing in your journal about your purpose in this wellness journey.

» Family and Friends

Family and friends can be one of the strongest reminders of our purpose. Today have a healthy meal with your family or some friends, and enjoy the social anchor that you have in your support system.

» Nutrition

Instead of a cooked appetizer, try putting out some sliced-up fruits and vegetables. Instead of a cream or mayonnaise-based dipping sauce (like French onion or ranch dressing), try serving hummus or baba ghanoush (roasted eggplant dip).

Evening Wrap-Up

From time to time, we must pause and remember our own purpose for being on the journey toward wellness. Our purpose keeps us anchored along the way. After the great flood in Genesis, God sent the rainbow as a reminder of the promise God made to Noah. But even now, the rainbow acts as a reminder of our covenant with God. It is a reminder of the larger picture and God's action in our lives. The rainbow anchors us on our life's journey. Today we need to remember the rainbows for our wellness journey.

"I will remember my covenant between me and you and all living creatures of every kind. . . . Whenever the rainbow appears in the clouds, I will see it and remember the everlasting covenant between God and all living creatures of every kind on the earth."

GENESIS 9:15–16

God of life, help me to remember my purpose as I continue on my journey. I pray that You would grant me rainbows to anchor me. In Your holy name, Amen.

Morning Reflection

As we strive to become healthy, changes are inevitable. In fact, change is not just a side effect of the journey—it is the point! But change, even change that we want, comes with its share of challenges. A great deal of change happening all at once can throw us off kilter. We can lose touch with our center and forget which way is "up." So today we will focus on how to keep our balance in the midst of all this change.

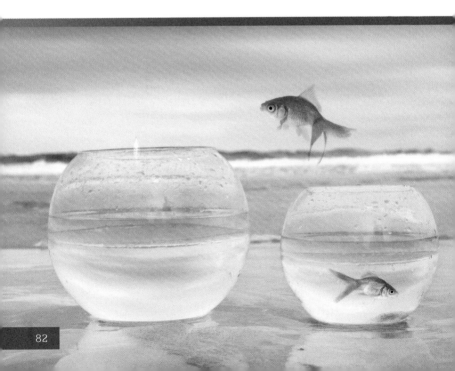

»Faith Life

Do you have a Bible verse or a special prayer that helps you to anchor your faith life? Today spend ten minutes and reflect on that one verse or prayer that "anchors" you, even as you have been on this journey full of change.

....

....

....

....

....

....

....

....

{ Change is not just a side effect of the journey— it is the point! }

PSALM 23

The LORD, the Psalmist's Shepherd.

A Psalm of David.

THE LORD is my ashepherd,
I shall bnot want.
2 He makes me lie down in agreen pastures;
He leads me beside lbquiet waters.
3 He crestores my soul;
He bguides me in the lcpaths of righteousness
For His name's sake.

»Medical

Your physician cannot treat what you do not tell her or him. Make sure that if you have any concerns, you tell your doctor. Doctors have heard (and seen) it all, so do not risk your health because you are feeling embarrassed.

....

....

»Movement

When you go to the grocery store, once you have loaded up your cart, take an extra walk around the store. It won't take you much time, and it will add another hundred or so steps to your day (depending on the size of your grocery store).

....

....

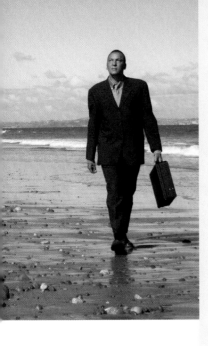

» Work

When work becomes topsy-turvy, it can be very easy to stress-eat without even recognizing what you are doing. Today if you start to feel overwhelmed at work, don't head for the vending machines; head for the door! Take a short break outside, breathe in some fresh air, and let your body relax before getting back to work.

» Emotional

How have you dealt with change in the past? Have you been able to embrace change? Or do you usually resist change? Go for a walk today, and take a different route than you usually do. Reflect on how you feel when you are trying something different.

» Family and Friends

Do your friends and family help anchor you? Let them know how important they are to you today. Write them a note, e-mail, or text message, or just call them up on the phone.

» Nutrition

Salads are definitely healthy, but be careful with the dressing and cheese! Use low-fat cheese, and substitute cream-based or mayonnaise-based dressings (like Ranch or Thousand Island) for a vinaigrette or even just some vinegar and oil with a little pepper and oregano.

Evening Wrap-Up

Change happens inevitably in life.

When it does eventually occur, change is very challenging, even when we are not actively changing multiple aspects of our lives. So, when we are trying to make changes in our lives, it can feel like running around without an anchor. The letter to the Hebrews reminds us that all things change—everything in the earth will fall away, and the earth itself will wear out. But God is constant and unchanging.

"In the beginning, Lord, you laid the foundations of the earth, and the heavens are the work of your hands. They will perish, but you remain; they will all wear out like a garment. You will roll them up like a robe; like a garment they will be changed. But you remain the same, and your years will never end."

HEBREWS 1:10–12

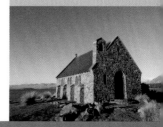

Dear Lord, thank You for Your constancy and Your unchanging love and support. Today in the midst of change, remind me that You are my anchor. In Your holy name, Amen.

Morning Reflection

At the end of this week, we are halfway through

the six weeks. Sometimes at the halfway point, we can feel both excited and discouraged. We might be able to see progress, and we may also look ahead and feel that we still have much more progress to make. It is easy now to run out of steam or to lose momentum. We are in the middle of the race, and it is now that we need to dig deep and tap into our extra stores of endurance to continue on the journey.

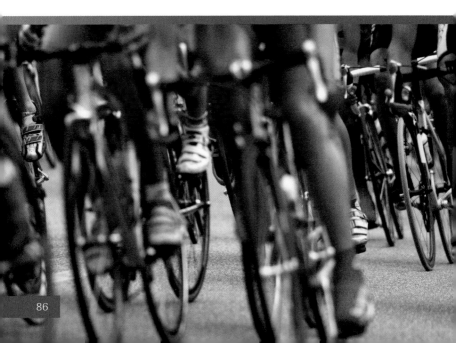

»Faith Life

Endurance requires, among other things, concentration. Today spend five minutes sitting quietly. Reflect on the journey till now and how God has been present with you.

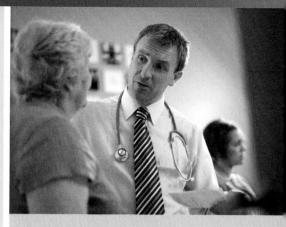

»Medical

Keep in mind that quick fixes in medicine are generally not a good long-term solution. The next time you have a doctor's appointment, talk to your care provider about your long-term health goals.

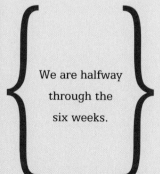

We are halfway through the six weeks.

»Movement

To build endurance, you need to occasionally push your limits. Today do as many jumping jacks as you can, take a one-minute break, and then do it again. Try that three times throughout the day.

»Work

Do you notice a time of day when you get hungry? Do you crave a specific food when you take your break? This may be habitual eating. Today when you feel hungry at work, drink some water or snack on some carrot sticks instead of heading for the donuts or vending machines.

»Emotional

Marathon runners will tell you that endurance is at least as emotional as it is physical. Today spend five minutes concentrating on breathing and repeat to yourself that you can continue on this journey. Try not to tell yourself that this is something that you cannot do.

»Family and Friends

Who is your oldest friend? Sometimes the relationships we have had the longest are the easiest to neglect. Take time today to think of a long-term friend whom you have not spoken to in a while and drop him or her a line.

»Nutrition

Tonight for dessert, make fruit kabobs and serve them with some low-fat yogurt or cottage or ricotta cheese instead of making a sugar-rich and fatty desert.

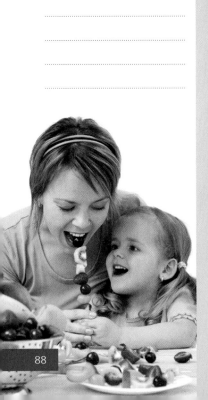

Evening Wrap-Up

The journey to wellness is a long one.

It is, in fact, a lifelong journey. We can easily run out of steam, particularly in the midst of a setback. Today we are halfway to the end of our six-week journey, but as far as we have come, we still have that far to go. And that can be intimidating and perhaps a bit unsettling. But in his letter to the Colossians, Paul reminds us that God gives us endurance and strength when we most need it.

May you be made strong with all the strength that comes from his glorious power, and may you be prepared to endure everything with patience, while joyfully giving thanks to the Father, who has enabled you to share in the inheritance of the saints in the light. He has rescued us from the power of darkness and transferred us into the kingdom of his beloved Son.

COLOSSIANS 1:11–13
NRSV

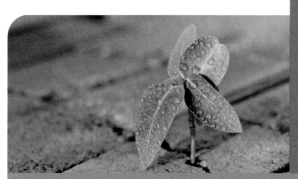

Enduring God, give me strength and endurance to continue on this journey, even when I have a setback. In Your name, Amen.

Rev. Clark has learned a lot about how his faith and health are connected.

He knew well the value of having an active faith life, but it was in following the advice of his doctor that he began to see the value of living a healthier life. As the weight came off—107 pounds in all—his energy level and stamina increased.

"I was dying too early," said Rev. Clark. "I was on six medications, I was overweight, and I was tired every day. I was in so much pain from being out of shape." He even began using a cane to get around his house.

Now, five years later, he exercises every day and not only feels better physically, but he believes that being healthier helps him care for his congregation better.

"The scripture I always use to motivate the members of my church is from Isaiah 37, about children coming to the point of birth but there's no strength to deliver them," he said. "I'm a charismatic preacher, and before, I'd come to a time when I needed to be there for people, to help carry them through difficult times, and physically I just couldn't do it. I was too tired! My members will tell you what a difference exercise has made. Now I can preach two to three hours without stopping!"

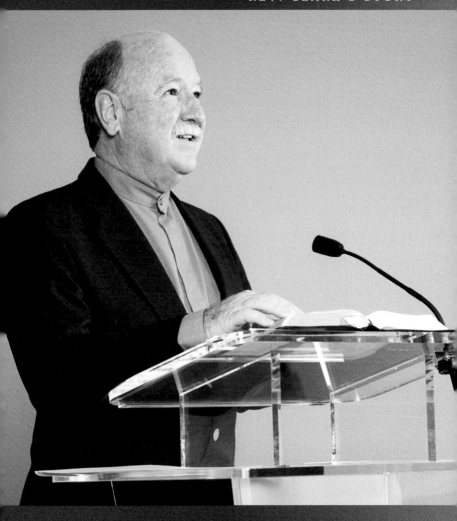

"I was dying too early," said Rev. Clark.

Optimal Health

Morning Reflection

Rev. Clark found out that an important part of wellness is learning to care for God's creation. Our wellness is intimately tied up in our relationship to God's creation. After all, we are a part of creation. We are created by God and are given a responsibility to care for God's creation. So living a wellness-oriented life is an act of stewardship—a way of caring for God's creation. This week, as we continue on our wellness journey, we will focus on how God's creation can be an important part of wellness.

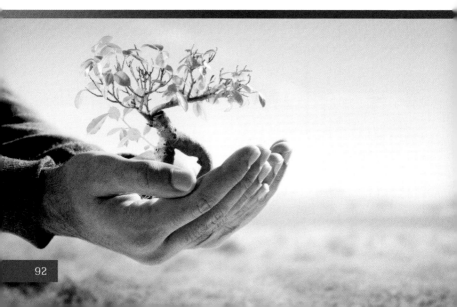

»Faith Life

All of creation belongs to God, though it can be easy to forget that. Today go for a prayerful walk and remember that the air you breathe and the ground you walk on belong to God.

{
Living a wellness-oriented life is an act of stewardship— a way of caring for God's creation.
}

»Medical

Good medicine is preventative medicine. This week we will focus on how to practice good preventative medicine at home. Today, make a list of the ways that you take care of yourself on a weekly or monthly basis.

»Movement

A wonderful way to get some exercise and appreciate God's creation is to go for a hike. Find a park in your area that has some trails available to hike. Don't forget to bring water and a healthy snack.

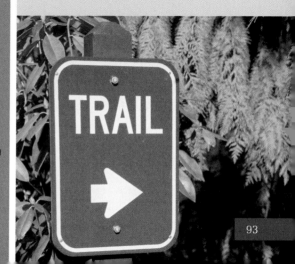

TRAIL

»Work

Being trapped inside all day can lead to some considerable burnout if you don't take time outside at some point. Today before work or after work, find five minutes to spend outside.

»Emotional

Today, practice slow, deep breathing. Relax your shoulders, lift your chin, close your eyes, and take a deep breath using your abdominal muscles. Hold your breath in for three seconds, and then slowly let your breath out.

»Family and Friends

Picnics are a wonderful way to connect with your family and friends. Today go on a picnic with your friends and family. Instead of hot dogs and hamburgers, pack fresh fruit, lean meats, and low-fat cheeses.

»Nutrition

This week we are going to focus on how to make your calories count. The first step is to eat whole grains. Buy whole-grain, low-fat breads, and pasta. Use brown rice instead of white rice.

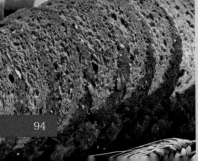

Evening Wrap-Up

We know that God is great. God made everything that we see, hear, and taste. But much of God's creation needs our care. We care for animals, oceans, the air, and the land in many different ways. But even when we fully acknowledge our responsibility for God's creation, we neglect that part with which we are the most intimately connected—ourselves! We regularly neglect God's creation by making poor nutritional decisions and not exercising. But we are moving toward better stewardship for all of God's creation.

O LORD my God, you are very great. . .
You stretch out the heavens like a tent, you set the beams of your chambers on the waters, you make the clouds your chariot, you ride on the wings of the wind, you make the winds your messengers. . . .
You set the earth on its foundations, so that it shall never be shaken.

PSALM 104:1–5 NRSV

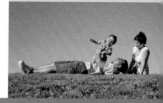

God of Creation, thank You for making the world and everything in it. Help me today to care for Your creation. In Your holy name, Amen.

Morning Reflection

Most of us spend most, if not all, of our time indoors. As a result, many of us lose touch with God's creation. In particular, we lose touch with the sun. The sun is very important to our health. Healthy exposure can lift our mood and give us more energy. Unhealthy exposure can lead to many skin problems, among them cancer. So knowing how to interact with the sun is very important on the journey to wellness.

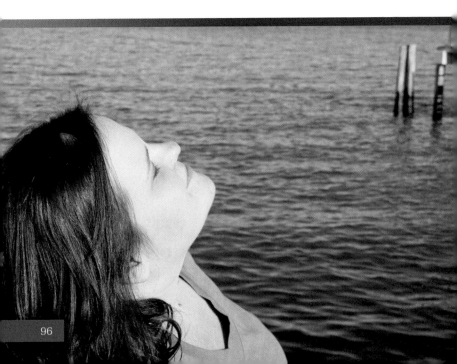

»Faith Life

When you walk out into the sun, do you think of God? Today when you have the sun in your eyes or you walk outside into the sunshine, say a brief prayer. "Thank You, God, for the sunshine."

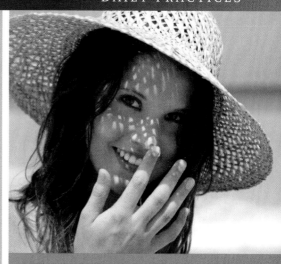

»Medical

Overexposure to the sun can cause serious health problems. Today check your body for moles and spots, using the ABCD rule. If the mole is Asymmetric, has irregular Borders, has a variation in Color, or has a Diameter larger than a pencil eraser, you should get it checked by your health care provider.

{ The sun is very important to our health. }

»Movement

Spend some time outside today—walking, or even going for a light jog. Remember to put on sun block before you spend any significant amount of time outside.

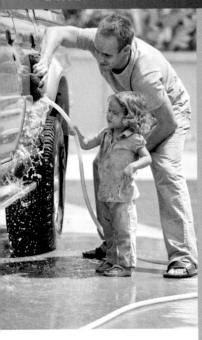

» Work

Enjoying the sun can be particularly difficult at our jobs, but our work is not just at our job. Today do some work outside. Wash your car, mow your lawn, or work in your garden.

» Emotional

The sun can provide a much-needed emotional lift, as well as vitamin D. Today find ten minutes to sit outside in the sun and practice deep breathing. Feel the sun's warmth, and try to let your body relax as you sit.

» Family and Friends

How often do you gather your family and friends for any kind of outdoor activity? Plan an outdoor social activity with your family and friends, even if it is only eating dinner outside.

» Nutrition

Do you eat cereal in the morning? Instead of a sweetened cereal, choose an unsweetened, whole grain cereal and sweeten it with cut fruit, such as bananas or berries. If you must have your cereal sweetened further, use an artificial sweetener.

Evening Wrap-Up

God created the sun, giving us a great gift and a great responsibility in it. We know that too much and the wrong kind of sun exposure can be detrimental to our overall health. However, too often we are so busy we forget to step into the light at all! Instead, we should be enjoying the wonders of God's creation. The truly amazing thing is, if we do enjoy God's creation responsibly, we will also be healthier. Enjoying the sunshine responsibly will make us healthier.

And God said, "Let there be light," and there was light. God saw that the light was good, and he separated the light from the darkness. God called the light "day," and the darkness he called "night." And there was evening, and there was morning— the first day.

GENESIS 1:3–5

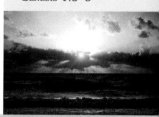

Joyful God, help me today to make the most of Your creation. Especially help me to enjoy the light that you have given me. In Your holy name, Amen.

Morning Reflection

If there is a part of God's creation that we all take for granted, it is probably the air. Our bodies breathe without our even thinking about it. Generally, we only notice the air if it smells bad or if there is not enough of it. But the air is a beautiful and important part of God's creation. So today we are going to focus on ways to be healthier using the air.

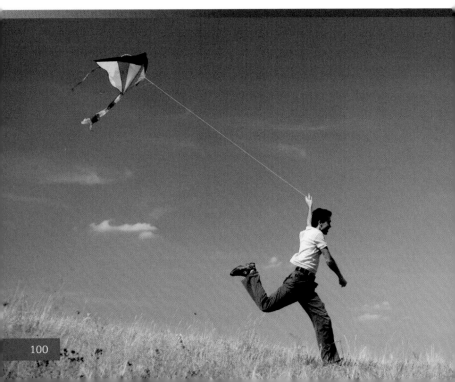

» Faith Life

There are dozens of verses in the Bible about how God uses the wind. Today read John 3:8, and when you encounter the wind today, take it as a reminder of God's Spirit moving in the world.

» Medical

Cigarette smoking greatly inhibits your ability to breathe. If you do smoke, talk to your primary care provider about ways to help you quit. Smoking simply does not have a place in wellness.

» Movement

When you walk, do you walk fast enough to feel the wind on your face or hair? Try scattering some "walking sprints" throughout your walk. This will help you to get your heart rate up, and you'll get more out of your walk.

» Work

If you feel anxiety at work, try to do some deep breathing. Breathe in through your nose and out through your mouth. You do not need to do this for extended periods of time at work. Simply give yourself a few breaths to relax.

» Emotional

Air is a very important part of stress relief. Today spend five minutes sitting with your back straight, breathing. Breathe in through your nose and out through your mouth.

» Family and Friends

Today go on a walk with a friend or family member. Concentrate on your breathing, and try to enjoy the fresh air.

» Nutrition

Avoid vegetables that are fried or prepared in heavy cream sauces or butter. Instead, bake your vegetables (such as squash and potatoes) or steam them (broccoli, asparagus, and green beans).

And God said,
"Let there be a vault
between the waters
to separate water
from water." So God
made the vault and
separated the water
under the vault from
the water above it.
And it was so.
God called the vault
"sky." And there was
evening, and there
was morning—
the second day.

GENESIS 1:6–8

Evening Wrap-Up

Like the sun, the air is a significant part of God's creation. We can feel

when it is not present. How many of us have breathed a sigh of relief on a hot day when a breeze breaks the heat just a little? Air—breath—is truly that which gives us life. But it often goes unnoticed. So today is a perfect day to stop and take notice of God's wonder in the creation of air.

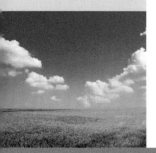

Lord, my God, thank You for giving me breath. Help me today to slow down and notice the gift and the beauty of the very air that I breathe. In Your name, Amen.

Morning Reflection

Water covers about 70 percent of the earth's surface.

Our own bodies are made up of 57 percent water on average. So it is safe to say that water is an important part of creation. But most health experts make it fairly clear that, generally speaking, we are not drinking enough water. The path to wellness is paved with water. And so today we will focus on the significant role that water plays in our wellness journey.

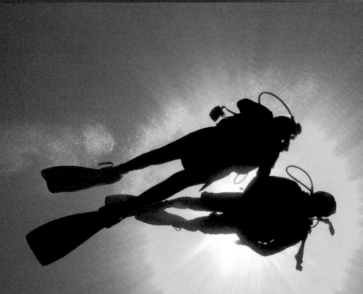

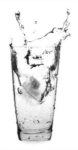

»Medical

Obesity tends to reduce the percentage of water in your body, which means that if you are overweight, you should be drinking even more water. Today count the glasses of water (or clear, unsweetened fluid) that you drink. You should be drinking about eight 8-ounce glasses a day.

»Movement

Swimming is excellent exercise. It is gentle on your joints and works just about every muscle group in your body. Today if you have access to a pool, go for a swim. Even spending ten minutes in the water will give you some great exercise.

»Faith Life

How often have we complained when it starts raining? Today write a prayer thanking God for the rain and for all of the ways that you are thankful for water in your life.

{ The path to wellness is paved with water. }

»Work

Bring a refillable water bottle to work.
When you are feeling thirsty or craving a
soda, fill up your water bottle and sip from
the bottle throughout the day. Staying hydrated will help you keep your energy levels
up and will keep you from drinking sugary
sodas.

»Emotional

Most of us shower in the morning. Today
take a five-minute shower at the end of the
day to warm your muscles and relax.

»Family and Friends

**Serving water with meals is a great way
to meet your daily water goals
(at least eight 8-ounce glasses).**
Today serve water instead of soda or other
sweetened beverages.

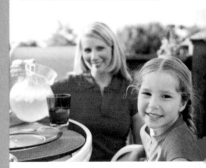

»Nutrition

**If you want a beverage other than
water, drink some unsweetened herbal
tea or fruit juice, but stick with 100
percent fruit juice.** Also, try to get more of
your fruit servings every day from whole fruit
rather than juice.

And God said, "Let the water under the sky be gathered to one place, and let dry ground appear." And it was so. God called the dry ground "land," and the gathered waters he called "seas." And God saw that it was good.

GENESIS 1:9–10

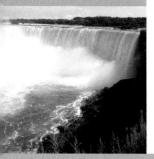

Evening Wrap-Up

God created the earth and made water a significant part of the earth

and of our lives. Throughout scripture we hear about water, both through the lack of water as in 1 Kings 17, and in the form of flood, as with Noah. Water is powerful, and God's power is reflected in water. It is no wonder that we are created of mostly water. So on this journey to wellness, we can remember that God's power—the power of water—is within us.

Creator of all things, today help me to remember that You created the earth and me as mostly water. Help me to remember that water is an important part of my journey to wellness. In Your holy name, Amen.

Morning Reflection

This week we have been reflecting on particular aspects of God's creation. Today we will focus on one area that we are working to transform on this journey—our bodies. If there is one aspect of God's creation that most of us have neglected and taken for granted, it is our own bodies. But God cares about our bodies, even to the extent that God became human in the person of Jesus Christ. When we forget that, it is only to our detriment.

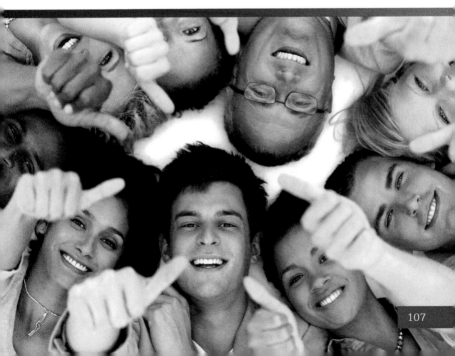

» Faith Life

Today at the time when you pray, pray a movement prayer. Stretch out your arms. Touch your toes. Stretch your neck. Feel the brilliance in God's creation and the way that your body is put together.

» Medical

If you do not give yourself a monthly breast exam or testicular exam, today is the day to start. Finding breast cancer and testicular cancer early greatly increases the chances of recovery.

» Movement

Today go for a brisk walk, and when you are finished, spend at least five minutes stretching. Try to feel and stretch as many muscles in your body as possible.

» Work

Work often requires repeating the same motion over and over again. When you take a break, spend five minutes doing something completely different than what you usually do. For example, if you sit at a computer typing most of the day, stand up and do jumping jacks.

» Emotional

Our emotions are more tied up with our bodies than we usually realize. Today spend five minutes smiling, even if you do not feel like smiling. Chances are, you will feel a little better at the end of those five minutes.

» Family and Friends

Many of our self-esteem issues come from directing hatred toward our own bodies. Today ask friends or family members to tell you what they like about your body.

» Nutrition

Drink about two glasses of milk today. But instead of whole milk, drink low-fat milk (either 1-percent or skim). Two servings of low-fat dairy each day are an important part of a healthy diet.

Evening Wrap-Up

Any time we are prepared to dismiss the body as somehow unimportant, we should remember this passage from Luke. God came to us as a man in the person of Jesus Christ. He had a body that was just as much a body as any of our bodies. And, to add emphasis, after He died, He rose again in a body. Our relationship with God is very much tied to the physical body.

He said to them, "Why are you troubled, and why do doubts rise in your minds? Look at my hands and my feet. It is I myself! Touch me and see; a ghost does not have flesh and bones, as you see I have." When he had said this, he showed them his hands and feet.

LUKE 24:38–40

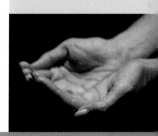

Incarnate God, thank You for this body that You have given me. Please help me to remember what a gift my body is, and help me as I strive to better care for myself. In Your holy name, Amen.

Morning Reflection

For the most part, we remember that God's creation includes things like the land and trees, and even our bodies (though an occasional reminder never hurts!). But something that we rarely think of as a part of God's creation is our community. We are created to be social beings, not isolated from one another. So today we will celebrate being a part of a community—a community that is a significant part of God's creation and of our wellness journey.

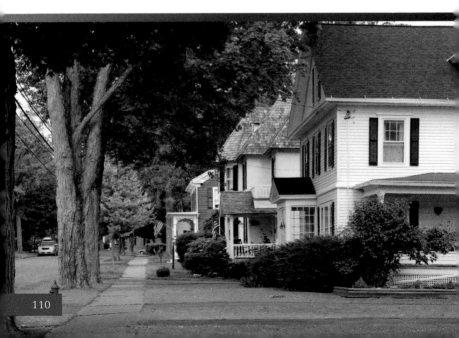

»Faith Life

Are you a part of a faith community, such as a church or a prayer group? Have you shared with them your journey to wellness? Today write the ways that your faith community is a part of your wellness journey.

»Medical

Know the signs of a heart attack: chest pain that feels like squeezing, pressure, or pain; pain or discomfort in the jaw, back, neck, arms, or stomach; shortness of breath; cold sweat and nausea or lightheadedness. Today brush up on the symptoms of major health events that could threaten your life or the life of someone you encounter.

»Movement

Housework burns calories and helps you feel like you've accomplished something. Today take on a task in your home that you don't usually do. For example, take out the trash, dust your bookshelves, clean the bathroom or the kitchen. Then invite someone over to enjoy your efforts!

> We are created to be social beings, not isolated from one another.

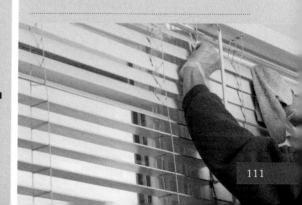

111

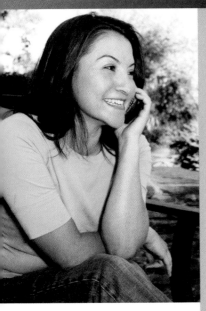

» Work

Do your coworkers know about your journey to wellness? Today tell at least one of your coworkers about your journey. Often workplaces can come together to strive toward wellness as a community.

» Emotional

Being a member of a community is a very important part of emotional wellness as well as physical wellness. Today instead of spending time writing in your journal, spend at least ten minutes sitting with someone who is a member of your support system and talk to them.

» Family and Friends

Do your family and friends make you laugh? Laughter is a wonderful way to burn calories and generally lift your mood. Today when spending time with friends or family, let yourself laugh freely.

» Nutrition

When "low-fat," "reduced-sugar," and "light" versions of your staple foods are available, choose them over the full-fat, full-sugar versions. That way you will dedicate more calories to important nutrients rather than "fillers" such as fats and sugars.

Evening Wrap-Up

We were not created to exist alone.

Instead, we have been created to be part of a community. In this passage from Acts, we see that early Christians ate together, worshiped together, and grew in faith together. Their wellness was intertwined with their community. Likewise, our wellness today is not only for us, but is for our community as well. As we continue on this journey, not only is God always with us, but we have companions in our faith communities, in our families, and even in our work communities.

Every day they continued to meet together in the temple courts. They broke bread in their homes and ate together with glad and sincere hearts, praising God and enjoying the favor of all the people. And the Lord added to their number daily those who were being saved.

ACTS 2:46–47

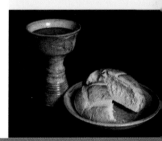

God of relationship, help me to reach out and open up to the communities of which I am a part. Help me to share my journey to wellness with them. In Your holy name, Amen.

113

Morning Reflection

We have reached the final day of our fourth week.

And as we have focused on the many aspects of God's creation, we have seen air, water, sun, and bodies. But we are left with one important aspect of God's creation that we also must care for: spirit. Though we often think of "health" as being primarily about the body, our spirits are central to wellness. Today we will focus on how our spirits contribute to our overall wellness.

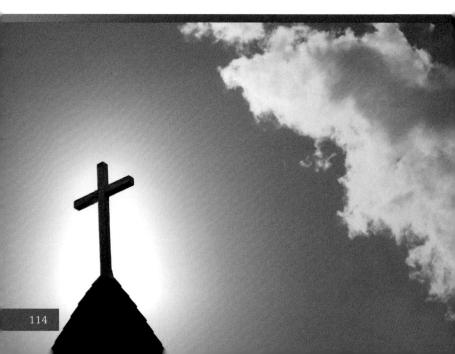

»Faith Life

What do you think a healthy spirit is? Today take ten minutes to pray and then write a few sentences about what a healthy spirit means to you.

....

....

....

....

....

....

....

....

....

....

{ Today we will focus on how our spirits contribute to our overall wellness. }

»Medical

File this piece of information away in your mind: If you have wounds, they should heal more or less within a week. If you have wounds, particularly on your legs and feet, that are not healing, you should see your primary care provider.

....

»Movement

Helping out a neighbor to do yard work or even to move is a wonderful act of kindness and generosity, and it can get your heart rate up and burn calories, to boot! Today try to help a friend, family member, or neighbor with a project.

....

....

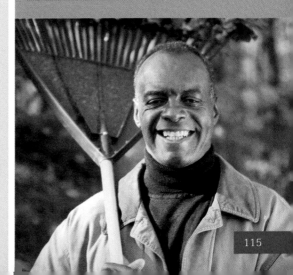

115

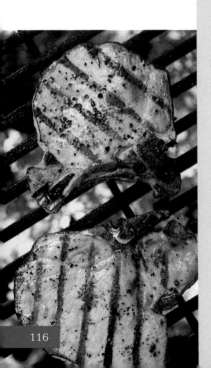

»Work

If you find yourself standing in one place for a period of time (making copies, talking on the phone, waiting for lunch to heat up), spend that time raising yourself onto your toes and then lowering yourself back down, increasing the strength in your calves.

»Emotional

We often expect perfection of ourselves. The trouble with such expectations is that we are simply not perfect, and we can become demoralized. Today write for ten minutes about a time that you have intentionally or inadvertently expected perfection from yourself.

»Family and Friends

Today recruit some family members and friends to help you with a project that you have been putting off—rearranging furniture, painting a room, mowing the lawn. Getting things accomplished is a great way to bond and lift spirits generally.

»Nutrition

When you cook meat, trim the visible fat before you cook it. Do not fry the meat— bake it or grill it. When it is cooked, drain the remaining fat.

Evening Wrap-Up

At this point in our journey, often we can start to notice a difference in our day-to-day lives. Perhaps we are not reaching as quickly for the bag of potato chips, or we are finding ways to add a few extra steps to each day. These changes may seem small, but they are, when added together, significant steps on the wellness journey. In his letter to the Galatians, Paul reminds us of the fruit of the Spirit. On our journey, the fruit of the Spirit that we are seeing are those extra steps.

By contrast, the fruit of the Spirit is love, joy, peace, patience, kindness, generosity, faithfulness, gentleness, and self-control. There is no law against such things. And those who belong to Christ Jesus have crucified the flesh with its passions and desires. If we live by the Spirit, let us also be guided by the Spirit.

GALATIANS 5:22–25
NRSV

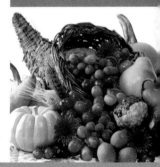

Dear Lord God, *help me to see Your Spirit at work in me as I continue on this journey to wellness.* In Your holy name, Amen.

Kathy's involvement in helping people to get moving

Kathy's involvement in helping people to get moving was born during her years as a middle school teacher at Lincoln Junior High School. In an effort to raise money to fight hunger in Memphis, she convinced students to walk with her; their initial efforts raised over three hundred dollars. She continued to motivate students to get moving during her time at Melrose High and Dunbar Elementary School.

Kathy continued to get more people moving by organizing neighborhood walks in her area. At the same time, she developed an interest in basketball through her husband's involvement with youth league basketball. She admits that she knew nothing about basketball prior to his coaching, but she was a fast learner.

The drive to get people moving became more personal when her husband suffered a major heart attack and was given five years to live. Following his heart surgery, her daily care for him taught her the science of healthy living. His doctors were amazed at his progress prior to his death. Her efforts in exercise and nutrition extended his life for many years.

Kathy took her exercise habits to another level by entering the Tennessee Senior Olympics. Her passion for running and basketball won her gold and silver medals in the three-mile run, the 100-meter dash, and the basketball free throw. She continued to stay active in community events through participation in many local races.

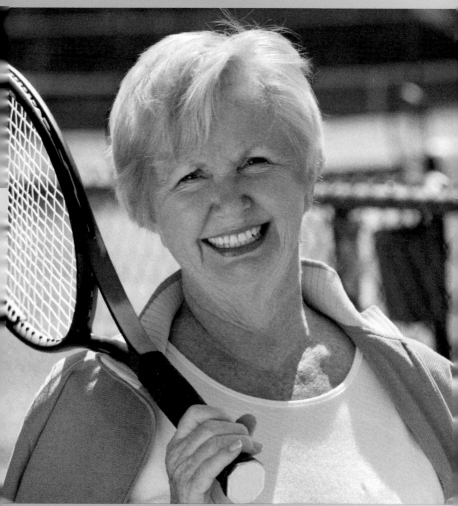

Her efforts in exercise and nutrition
extended her husband's life for many years.

Optimal Health

Morning Reflection

The journey to wellness is not a one-path-fits-all journey. Sometimes, as with Kathy's story, we might begin on what we consider to be the path, and we end up looking at something different than what we expected. Kathy started on a journey to feed children and ended up winning the 100-meter dash! This week we will be considering the variety of directions our journeys might take us. In particular, we will focus on the fact that the journey is infinitely varied.

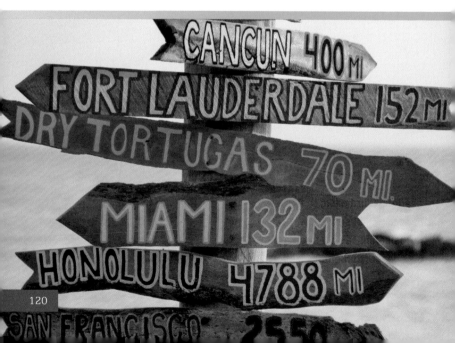

»Faith Life

Our faith journey, like our wellness journey, is a long and varied one. Spend ten minutes today writing about a time in your faith journey when you thought you were beginning one particular stage of a journey but ended up somewhere else entirely.

{ The journey is infinitely varied. }

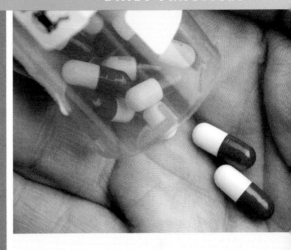

»Medical

Are you on medications? Have you been feeling better? Do not stop taking any medications until you have discussed it with your primary care provider. Stopping medication suddenly can lead to relapse, drug resistance, or unexpected side effects.

»Movement

Go for a walk in your neighborhood today. Take a coin, and each time you arrive at a corner, flip the coin to decide whether to turn left or right.

121

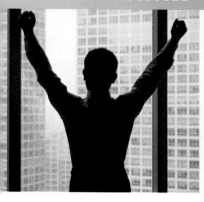

»Work

Each hour at work, take a minute or two just to stretch your arms and back. This will help keep you limber and can help keep you focused throughout the day.

»Emotional

The unpredictability of our wellness journey can sometimes feel overwhelming. Today make a list of what your expectations are at this point in your journey. Compare them with your expectations at the beginning of the journey.

»Family and Friends

Family and friends can be our constants when other things in life are unpredictable. Today make a healthy meal for your family or some friends. Enjoy the food, but focus on the company and conversation.

»Nutrition

When you are trying to cut out sugar, add lemon, orange, or lime zest to a recipe. The citrus zest will add flavor and interest to a dish, so you will be less likely to miss the sugar.

Evening Wrap-Up

Even with the most extensive planning, we cannot know where the journey will take us. This passage from James reminds us that we cannot count our plans as guaranteed. Sometimes plans change and paths wander in unexpected directions. But this should not halt our journey. Instead, it should drive us to be ever more dependent on God's grace along the way.

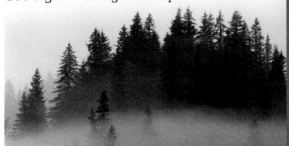

Now listen, you who say, "Today or tomorrow we will go to this or that city, spend a year there, carry on business and make money." Why, you do not even know what will happen tomorrow. What is your life? You are a mist that appears for a little while and then vanishes. Instead, you ought to say, "If it is the Lord's will, we will live and do this or that."

JAMES 4:13–15

Guiding God, thank You for the journey that You have laid out for me. Help me today to embrace the journey, whatever direction it takes me. In the name of Your Son, Amen.

Morning Reflection

As we continue on the journey to wellness, we will inevitably have a variety of new experiences: new foods, new ways to move, and new habits. This is a part of the journey. These experiences can be exciting, terrifying, exhausting, or all of the above. What we must always try to remember is that God is with us as we have those experiences. In a word, God is with us on this journey.

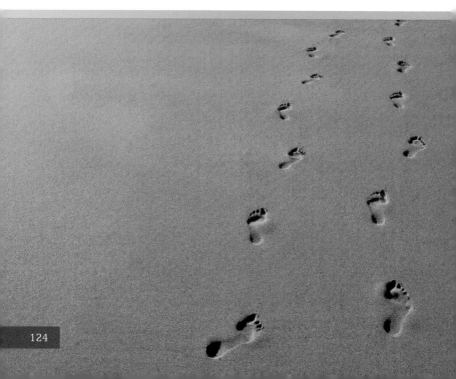

»Faith Life

Today each time you eat, give thanks for the food that God has given you. Try to pause, even when you have a small snack, to say a prayer.

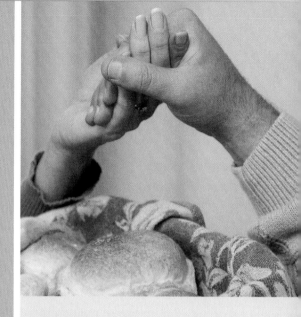

{ God is with us on this journey. }

»Medical

An important aspect of overall health is oral health. Today make sure that you have a dentist appointment scheduled. You should have a checkup and teeth cleaning every six months.

»Movement

Today spend fifteen minutes doing abdominal strength exercises. Standard sit-ups and crunches are a very good way to strengthen your core. Make sure that you do not strain your neck or back as you do those crunches!

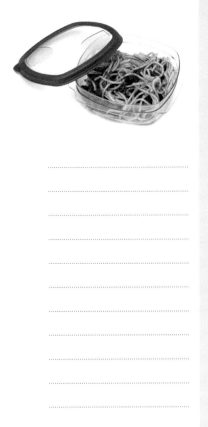

» Work

Instead of going out to eat or getting lunch out of a vending machine, bring in a lunch made from your leftovers from last night's dinner. It is almost guaranteed to be healthier, and it is much less expensive!

» Emotional

Give yourself a rest today. Spend a half hour doing something you really enjoy. Read a book, listen to music, watch a television show, or take a bath. Just take care of yourself without worrying about the things that you "have to do" for thirty minutes.

» Family and Friends

Do you have friends or family who are somehow involved in this journey with you? If you do not, make a list of potential friends or family members who might partner with you as you continue on the journey.

» Nutrition

Some fats are necessary for balanced nutrition. Healthy fats can be found in avocado, seeds and nuts, olive oil, and fish. Today prepare a meal using mostly healthy fats. (No fried food or butter.)

Evening Wrap-Up

As we form these new habits and have these new experiences, we need to remember many things. Among them is the knowledge that we are making *gradual* changes that are meant to end in *lifestyle* changes. But the changes that we are making are not all-or-nothing and they are not all-at-once. Instead, they are one new experience at a time, repeated until the new experiences become habit. As we go through these changes, we can taste and see the goodness of God, recognizing that in the midst of any new experience, we can take refuge in God.

I sought the LORD and he answered me; he delivered me from all my fears. Those who look to him are radiant . . . . Taste and see that the LORD is good; blessed is the one who takes refuge in him.

PSALM 34:4–5, 8

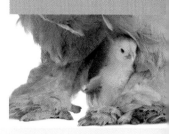

Lord God, thank You for the gift of new experiences. Help me to take refuge in You when I feel overwhelmed by the newness. In Your holy name, Amen.

Morning Reflection

On our wellness journey, we encounter many different times and seasons. That is simply the nature of the journey. Just as our seasons change, we will experience periods of feeling very good and seasons of feeling not-so-good. But it is important that as we travel through these seasons, we do not give up on the journey altogether. Instead, we must recognize that seasons require patience and perseverance. Today we will concentrate on the seasons that make up the journey.

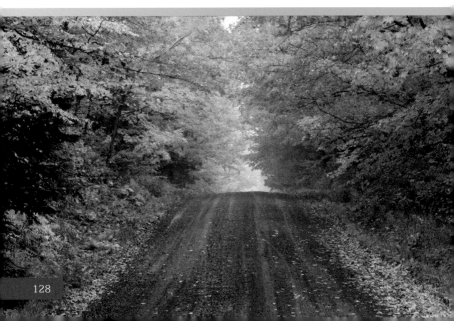

» Faith Life

What is your favorite season of the year? Spend five minutes writing about your favorite season. Then spend five minutes writing about your least favorite season. Can you find God in both your favorite and least favorite seasons?

» Medical

Today when you brush your teeth, time yourself. You should brush your teeth for about two minutes, spending thirty seconds brushing each quadrant (upper left, upper right, lower left, and lower right).

» Movement

Remember that you can walk outside whatever the season. Today go for a walk outside. If it is cold, wear a coat. If it is hot, wear shorts and a T-shirt. Try to enjoy the seasons that you experience.

» Work

Most workplaces have periods that are busy and periods that are slower. Whatever your work environment is like at this moment, find five minutes to breathe and stretch a little.

» Emotional

Are your expectations that your lifestyle changes will be all-or-nothing? Today take five minutes to write in your journal, reminding yourself that setbacks and individual "failures" are just seasons. If we persevere, they pass.

» Family and Friends

Ask one of the family members or friends on the list you made yesterday to be your "wellness buddy." Walking this journey without a partner can make a difficult journey even more difficult.

» Nutrition

Variety is the key to a balanced diet. Today prepare a meal that includes as many colors as you can fit into the meal. To easily add some variety, offer some raw, cut vegetables (such as carrot sticks or sliced red bell pepper) in addition to a cooked vegetable.

Evening Wrap-Up

He changes times and seasons; he deposes kings and raises up others. He gives wisdom to the wise and knowledge to the discerning. He reveals deep and hidden things; he knows what lies in darkness, and light dwells with him.

DANIEL 2:21–22

God has built times and seasons into creation.

Change is simply a part of the world that God has made. But that does not necessarily make the changes that we encounter easy, even when those changes are welcomed. We know that God can break through any resistance to change that might dwell deep in our psyche. After all, it is God who "gives wisdom to the wise."

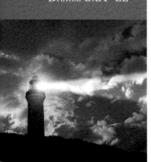

Loving Lord, help me to make healthy changes in my life as I move forward. I pray that You would break down the barriers in my mind, body, and spirit that keep me from being well. In Your holy name, Amen.

Morning Reflection

Our wellness journey consists of not just differing seasons, but also of many different sounds. Because the journey to wellness is about changing our entire lifestyle, it is only natural that some of the sounds that we hear on a regular basis will change over time. We may even find ourselves speaking differently about wellness and our bodies. After all, Kathy never expected that she would hear her friends cheering her on at the finish line of a race, but that is where her journey led her.

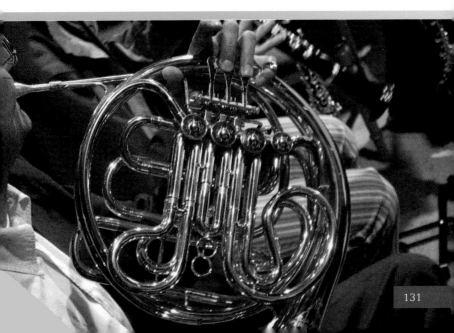

»Medical

Do you floss your teeth every day? If not, today is the day to begin. Floss your teeth after you brush before going to bed. If your teeth are spaced tightly together, buy floss that is wax coated.

»Movement

Sound can be an important part of movement, but we often ignore it. Today go for a walk and listen to the rhythm of your feet on the ground and the sound of your breath. You may even be able to hear your heartbeat as it rises.

»Faith Life

What is your favorite sound in the world? Today write for five minutes about that sound. What does the sound remind you of? Where does God fit into that sound?

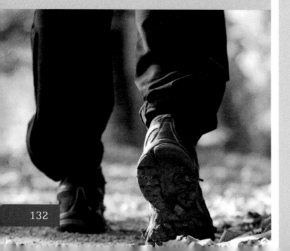

It is only natural that some of the sounds that we hear on a regular basis will change.

»Work

If you are able today, put on some soft music while you work, using either small speakers or headphones. Listening to music can help to pass time and can also lift your mood or relax you.

»Emotional

If you feel frustrated, try making some noise. Scream into a pillow or bang some pots and pans together. Making the noise will help you to relieve some aggression and frustration so that you can gradually relax.

»Family and Friends

When you gather family and friends for a holiday or special occasion, think about playing games instead of focusing entirely on food. That way the gathering is more about being in each other's company rather than eating.

»Nutrition

Instead of buying canned soup, make a large pot of soup on your stove top or in a slow cooker. Eat some tonight and put at least one night's worth in the freezer to eat on a busy day. (Hint: season the soup with spices and herbs rather than with salt.)

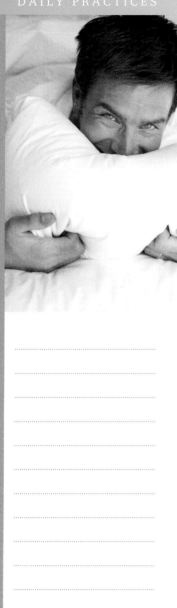

*Shout for joy to
God, all the earth!
Sing the glory of
his name; make
his praise glorious.
Say to God,
"How awesome
are your deeds! . . .
All the earth bows
down to you;
they sing praise
to you, they sing
the praises of
your name."*

PSALM 66:1–4

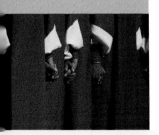

Evening Wrap-Up

Sound can be reminders of God's grace and presence in our lives.

Noises can also be ways that we can praise and worship God. The psalmist writes, "Make a joyful noise." Can there be a more joyful noise than a healthy person moving and enjoying the movement? What would happen if we considered the sound of our feet on the pavement on the same level as praise and worship songs? We would probably walk a little more. As we move forward, let us remember that God loves us and wants us to be healthy.

Dear God, thank You for the gift of sound. Help me to hear the music all around me, even in my own footsteps. In Your holy name, Amen.

Morning Reflection

As we continue on the wellness journey, the things we are used to seeing may begin to look different. Our eyesight, in a manner of speaking, changes. Food labels and methods of preparation that were once appealing may not be so appealing anymore. Riding the elevator may look like a wasted opportunity to take the stairs. Wellness changes our perspective in many ways. Today we will focus on the ways in which wellness changes our sight.

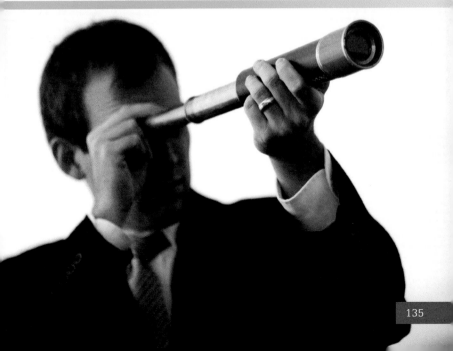

» Faith Life

Do you have potluck dinners at your church? The next time you have a potluck dinner, try bringing a healthy dish instead of a more typical dish. (For example, bring fresh fruit instead of a pie.)

» Medical

How is your vision? Are there things that give your sight trouble, either up close or far away? Today take a few minutes to critique your vision, and if necessary, make an appointment to have your eyes checked or your prescription updated.

» Movement

Go for a walk today. Walk for as long as you can manage and take in the sights of the world around you. Try to notice the difference in your walking now from when you started.

» Work

If it is flu season, get the flu shot. The workplace is a hotbed for the flu virus. (You should get a flu shot regardless, but particularly if you work at a place with lots of people, a shared bathroom, etc.)

» Emotional

Today for comparison's sake, keep a log of your emotions throughout the day. Write when you feel happy, tired, frustrated, or bored, and record what you do (if anything) to deal with the emotion.

» Family and Friends

Reaching out to family and friends when you need support can sometimes be difficult. But today let one of your friends or family members know what kind of support you need on your wellness journey, even if they are not on the journey with you.

» Nutrition

If you are craving something sweet, eat a piece of fruit. If you really want a piece of candy or a sugary desert, try eating a small piece of dark chocolate. Dark chocolate has less fat and less sugar than milk chocolate.

Evening Wrap-Up

Before we make an effort to live wellness-oriented lives, it can be like living in blindness. But as we make progress toward wellness, our eyes are opened and we can see both who we are and how God relates to us in this journey. After all, God opens the eyes of the blind. God is forever faithful, and as we continue on this journey, we can lean on God, giving ourselves over to God's grace.

Happy are those whose help is the God of Jacob, whose hope is in the LORD their God, who made heaven and earth, the sea, and all that is in them; who keeps faith forever; who executes justice for the oppressed; who gives food to the hungry. . . .
The LORD opens the eyes of the blind. The LORD lifts up those who are bowed down.

PSALM 146:5–8 NRSV

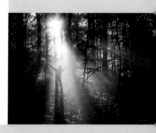

Faithful God, I know that You can help me change my wellness perspective. I pray today that You would help me to see the importance of this journey. In Your holy name, Amen.

137

Morning Reflection

This week we have been focusing on some of the fruit of our journey to this point. We are beginning to approach the end of our six-week journey, and so we are seeing some small results. But the true results will not really show themselves until we live our lives differently. That is the point of this journey: a changed life. Or rather, the point of the journey is not just a changed life, it is *life*. The fruit of wellness is life.

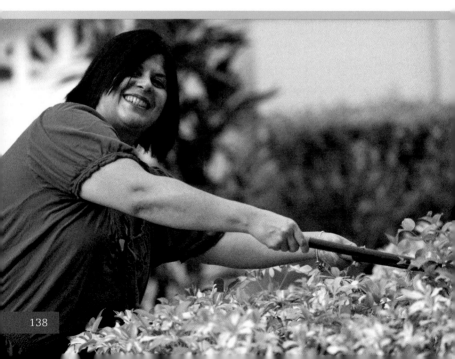

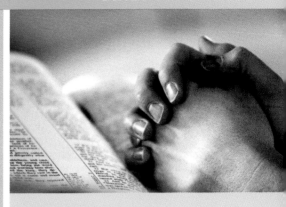

»Faith Life

Today spend five minutes meditating. Breathe deeply, quiet your "inner voices," and turn your focus to the wellness journey. Where have you felt God on the journey?

....

....

....

....

....

....

....

....

....

»Medical

Make a mental note: If you forget to take your medication for one dose, do not take a double dose. Instead, call your primary care provider and ask whether you should take a dose immediately or wait until it is time for the next dose to get back on track.

....

....

»Movement

Today work out your arms while you get some cardio exercise. Go for a walk and carry some light hand weights (two or five pounds—nothing heavier) with you. Do some bicep curls as you walk.

....

....

....

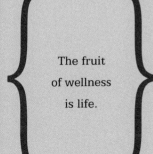

{ The fruit of wellness is life. }

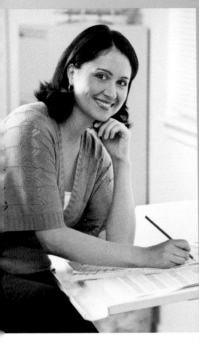

» Work

How has this journey impacted your work life thus far? Have you noticed changes in your attitude, your work ethic, your productivity? Consider how you have changed your work life today and take note of your improvements.

» Emotional

Take ten minutes and check in with your current emotional state. Do you feel good? Discouraged? Frustrated? Write about what you are feeling, particularly in relation to your wellness journey.

» Family and Friends

Today go out to a favorite restaurant with some friends and/or family. Again, try to enjoy the company and the socializing more than the food. Enjoy the food, but make the social interaction the star of the evening.

» Nutrition

Do not eat at the first sign of hunger. Instead, wait until you are experiencing strong feelings of hunger to eat, because when you start to get hungry, your body taps into your fat stores for energy.

Evening Wrap-Up

It is normal at this point in the journey to begin worrying about what will happen next. But it is important to realize that the small steps that we have been taking over the last five weeks have been adding up. We are making progress toward wellness. Each time we exercise or prepare a healthy meal, we take another step along the journey. Even setbacks are simply a part of the journey. And so it is not for us to worry but to continue on.

Then Jesus said to his disciples: "Therefore I tell you, do not worry about your life, what you will eat; or about your body, what you will wear. For life is more than food, and the body more than clothes. Consider the ravens: They do not sow or reap, they have no storeroom or barn; yet God feeds them. And how much more valuable you are than birds!"

LUKE 12:22–24

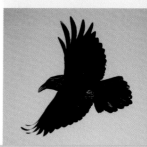

God of each new step, help me today to lay down my worry and to simply focus on the journey ahead. In Your holy name, Amen.

Morning Reflection

Today we reach the final day of the fifth week, Day 35. We are coming to the end of our six-week journey, but the larger journey is really just beginning. Think of Jesus' forty-day walk in the wilderness. It was preparation for the rest of His life, not His entire life. Our six-week journey is the preparation for the wellness journey after the six weeks are completed. The journey to wellness is a journey toward healing. Today we will focus on how wellness heals.

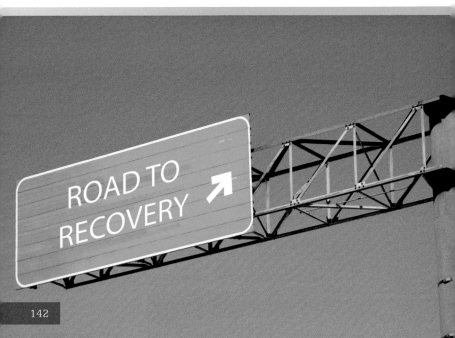

»Faith Life

Today read Luke 8:40–56. Then spend five minutes writing about when you have experienced God's healing grace in your life. Keep in mind, God heals in many different ways.

....
....
....
....
....
....
....
....
....
....

{ Our six-week journey is the preparation for the wellness journey after the six weeks are completed. }

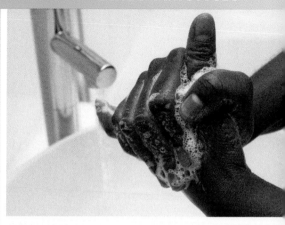

»Medical

One of the best ways to prevent both serious and minor illnesses (such as the common cold or staph infections) is to wash your hands frequently, particularly during times of the year when most people are inside. Also try keeping a bottle of alcohol-based hand-sanitizing gel with you.

»Movement

Exercise is incredibly healing, as we saw with Kathy's husband. Today spend ten minutes warming up your muscles with some jumping jacks or jogging in place. Then spend at least five minutes stretching your muscles.

....
....
....

» Work

Today at work, if you are stuck sitting for long periods of time, try to move your feet by bouncing your legs up and down or even rolling your ankles around. This will help maintain circulation in your legs and can help relieve pain or swelling that comes with sitting.

» Emotional

Physical healing means very little without emotional healing. Take ten minutes and write about a time in your life that you experienced emotional healing, such as a time when you have forgiven or been forgiven.

» Family and Friends

A large part of any healing is our support system. Today have a conversation with the members of your family and friends who are an important part of your support system. Tell them what healing on this journey looks like for you.

» Nutrition

Cheese is the number one source of saturated fat in the American diet. Today switch to a 2-percent milk cheese and pay attention to portion size. (One serving of cheese is one ounce, about the size of six dice.)

Evening Wrap-Up

We are on a journey toward wellness. As we walk this journey, we realize that it is also a journey of physical, emotional, and spiritual healing. As we wrap up this week, we look back on the ways that this journey is healing those parts of us that were not whole, and we can give thanks to God for that healing. As Isaiah reminds us, God can restore us to health and help us to live. God gives us strength for the journey even when we have a difficult time finding that strength for ourselves.

"Lord, by such things people live; and my spirit finds life in them too. You restored me to health and let me live."

ISAIAH 38:16

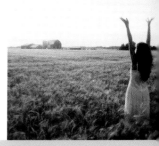

Healing God, thank You for walking this journey with me. Help my body to heal as I continue on my journey toward wellness. In Your holy name, Amen.

A little more than four years ago, Deb had a decision to make—start giving herself four insulin shots every day or change the way she was living.

"I told my doctor, 'Give me one month to exercise and lose twenty pounds so I can stay on oral medication.' " Her doctor agreed.

So she started to exercise. One month later, Deb had indeed lost the twenty pounds she set out to lose, and she had gained something even more important—confidence.

Since then, Deb has lost a total of 190 pounds and has reduced the number of prescription medications she takes from ten to two. She even participated in her first-ever 5K race.

Results like those take dedication and hard work, but if you ask Deb how she did it, she's quick to give credit to God.

"God said, 'If you take the first step, I'll do the rest,' and I said, 'God, I'm putting this in Your hands,' " Deb recalled. "I've been holding on for the ride ever since. When I look at how far God has brought me. . . Oh, thank You, Lord! I'm not fixin' to give up. And if I can do it, you can do it, but you can't do it for anyone but yourself. Don't do it for your family or anyone else. Do it for yourself."

Two years ago, Deb had a stroke. She survived. Her doctor told her that her regular exercise had likely saved her life.

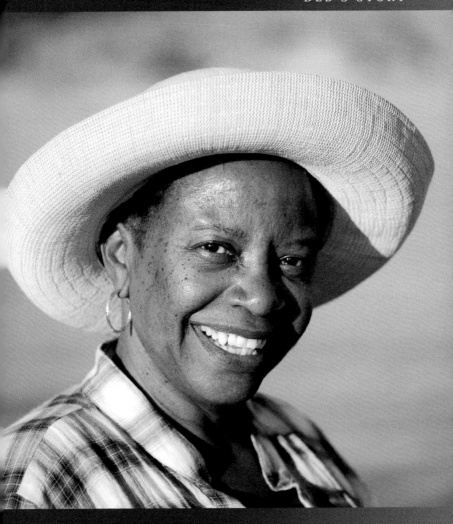

"Don't do it for your family or anyone else. Do it for yourself."

Morning Reflection

Some conversions happen quickly, as with Deb's wake-up call to change her life or go on insulin. Other conversions happen slowly and over longer periods of time. For most of us, our conversion stories are a combination of quick conversion and a longer journey. The journey to wellness is no different. We often have a singular moment when we realize that we must do something to live better. But it is only in the longer journey that we are actually changed.

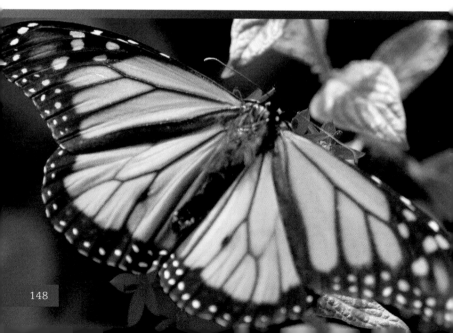

»Faith Life

Today try a walking meditation. Go for a slow walk around your neighborhood without a specific plan. Simply let yourself wander for about ten minutes. Try to quiet yourself and just walk.

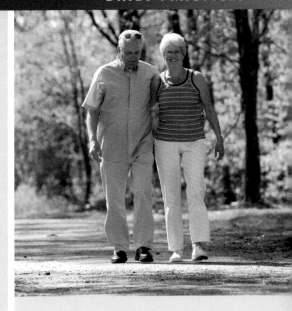

{ It is only in the longer journey that we are actually changed. }

»Medical

At this point in the journey, you may want to increase your exercise level. If you are going to engage in any kind of a rigorous exercise program, make sure that you talk to your doctor first. He or she can help you safely exercise.

»Movement

Getting regular exercise can lower your risk of diseases such as diabetes, heart disease, and arthritis. Today go for a walk, trying to raise your heart rate. Make sure that you breathe deeply as your heart rate rises.

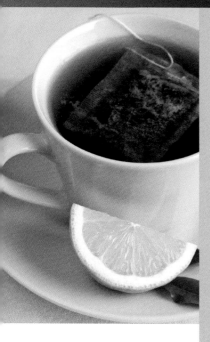

»Work

Bring a stash of decaffeinated, non-sweetened herbal teas into work. When you feel like drinking a cup of coffee, have a cup of herbal tea instead. That way you will be more hydrated, and you will avoid the bursts of energy and crashes that come with caffeine and sugar.

»Emotional

Many times, quick conversions are what we could call mountaintop experiences. But the real work is done in the valleys. Today write about times when you have been on the mountaintop and how those experiences translate to the work in the valleys.

»Family and Friends

Often, our family and friends are not on exactly the same path to conversion as us. Today if your family and friends do not seem to understand why you are on the journey, tell them your conversion story to help them understand where you are coming from.

»Nutrition

If you eat canned fruit instead of fresh fruit, rinse the fruit off before you eat it. This will wash away some of the excess sugar and syrup that the fruit comes in.

Evening Wrap-Up

We probably remember the story of Saul's conversion to Paul on the road to Damascus. But we so often focus on the moment when he fell off his horse instead of the long road that lay ahead of him. Paul's journey really began on the road to Damascus. Likewise, our conversion to wellness might begin with a bang, but like Paul's journey, it is in the individual steps and the long road ahead where the change actually happens.

As he neared Damascus on his journey, suddenly a light from heaven flashed around him. He fell to the ground and heard a voice say to him, "Saul, Saul, why do you persecute me?" "Who are you, Lord?" Saul asked. "I am Jesus, whom you are persecuting," he replied. "Now get up and go into the city, and you will be told what you must do."

Acts 9:3–6

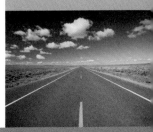

God of the journey, help me in both my moments of instantaneous conversion and on the long road ahead. In Your holy name, Amen.

Morning Reflection

As we continue on this journey, in many ways we are coming to know ourselves. After all, we are coming to know new limits and perhaps new attitudes. What we can also realize is that in this journey, we can begin to understand how God knows us as well. We can remember that God created us whole, and as we continue on the journey, we begin to know our whole self as well. Today we will try to see ourselves as God sees us.

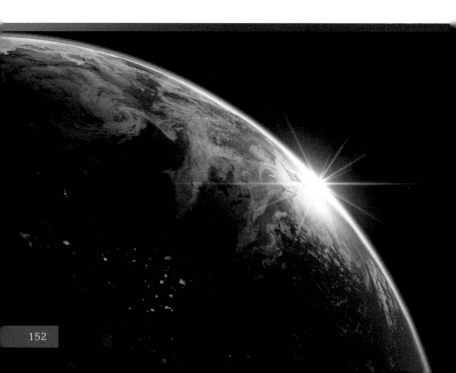

»Faith Life

The first step in "Love your neighbor as yourself" is to love yourself. Today spend five minutes writing about what it means to love yourself. Remember that God loves you.

....

....

....

....

....

....

....

....

....

{
Today we will try
to see ourselves
as God sees us.
}

»Medical

Before you start taking a vitamin or supplement, consult with your health care provider. Sometimes vitamins and supplements can have interactions with prescription medications that would not be listed on the bottle.

»Movement

Today spend ten minutes stretching and exploring all of the parts that God made. Touch your toes, cross your arms over your chest, roll your neck, stretch your arms up over your head, and stretch your back.

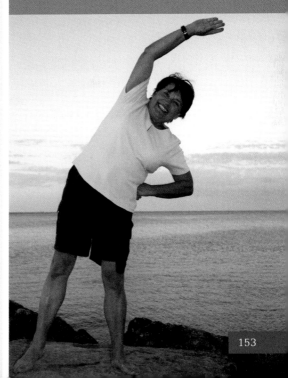

153

» Work

If you must go out for lunch at work, try to avoid eating fast food. Instead, try to find a place where you can order lean protein and vegetables that are not fried.

» Emotional

One of the keys to emotional wellness is to spend time engaged in self-care. Today write down one area in your life where you could use some more self-care. Do you need to find some extra alone time? Do you need to schedule more time with friends?

» Family and Friends

When you plan activities with your family and friends, try going to a park, playground, or museum instead of going immediately to a restaurant. This way you will have some kind of physical activity built into your outing.

» Nutrition

Know exactly what you are eating. When you go shopping, make sure to read the food label before you buy the food. The ingredients listed first are the major ingredients in that product.

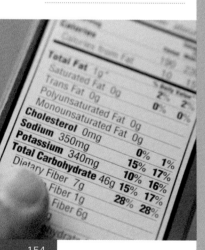

Evening Wrap-Up

When we go through times when we forget just how much God cares for us, remember Psalm 139. God knows every detail of our lives. God put each of us together, even as we grew in the womb. We could never have done anything to deserve such loving attention, and yet we are all "fearfully and wonderfully made."

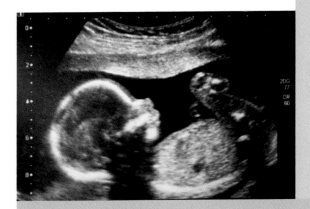

*You have searched me, L*ORD*, and you know me. You know when I sit and when I rise; you perceive my thoughts from afar. You discern my going out and my lying down; you are familiar with all my ways. . . . For you created my inmost being; you knit me together in my mother's womb. I praise you because I am fearfully and wonderfully made; your works are wonderful, I know that full well.*

PSALM 139: 1–3, 13–14

Dear Lord God, I know that I am fearfully and wonderfully made. Help me to remember the care with which I was brought into this world. In Your holy name, Amen.

Morning Reflection

As we approach the end of this six-week journey,

it is important for us to set up plans and support for the journey beyond these six weeks. After all, wellness is a lifelong journey. It is not a goal that can be attained and then left behind. Throughout the journey to this point, we have been working to put habits and lifestyle changes into place to prepare us for the next steps. Today we will begin thinking about what those next steps will be.

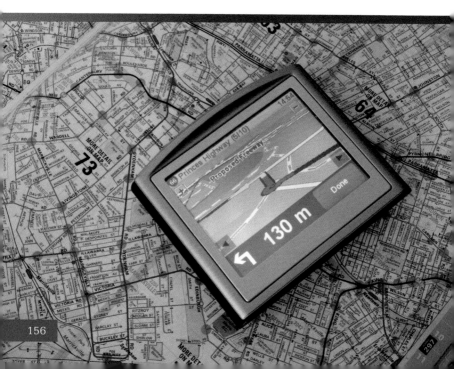

» Faith Life

Our faith can be an anchor for us when things become challenging. Today spend five minutes writing about the things, people, places, and activities that give you hope on your journey.

» Medical

If you are over fifty, have a conversation with your primary care provider about getting a colonoscopy. It is a procedure that can detect colon cancer, and the earlier colon cancer is detected, the better your chances at survival and recovery.

» Movement

If you run to the store to buy a gallon of milk, carry the milk with you instead of putting it in a cart. Then while you stand in line, do some alternating bicep curls with it.

» Work

Bring an insulated lunch bag to work with some raw chopped vegetables such as celery, carrots, and red bell peppers to snack on when you get hungry. If you want to add a little spice, throw in a few radishes as well.

» Emotional

Branching out into the next part of the journey can be intimidating. Today make a list of the activities that you have discovered that work to help you relieve your stress.

» Family and Friends

Your family and friends will be very important to your journey. Today try to set up a regular walking time with (at least) one of your friends or family members. Having a regular time will help you to get into (and stay in) the habit of walking.

» Nutrition

If you are tired of eating so many servings of vegetables each day (aim for three–five), try swapping out two servings of raw or cooked vegetables with ¾ cup of vegetable juice. Just be sure to account for added sugar in the juice.

Evening Wrap-Up

The journey from here forward is really about hope. We have the skills and knowledge that we need to be healthy. But what we need at this point is to continue on the journey, never ceasing in our hope that our lives can and do change. Peter reminds us that the hope that God gives us is always the hope for new life through the resurrection of Jesus Christ.

Praise be to the God and Father of our Lord Jesus Christ! In his great mercy he has given us new birth into a living hope through the resurrection of Jesus Christ from the dead, and into an inheritance that can never perish, spoil or fade.

1 PETER 1:3–4

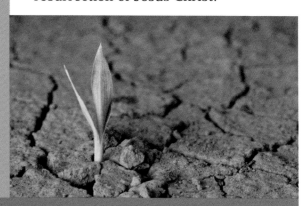

Gracious God, help me today as I begin to look down the road. Grant me hope and encouragement for what is to come. In Your holy name, Amen.

Morning Reflection

As we approach the final stretch of our six-week journey, we need to be reminded that we are not alone on the journey. Though it is true that we are, in most cases, trying to change individual habits, the people who surround us can give us encouragement. Furthermore, encouraging others on the wellness journey can help us to feel encouraged ourselves. Today we will focus on ways that we can surround ourselves with fellow travelers on the journey.

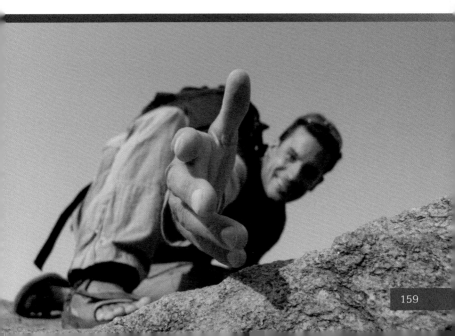

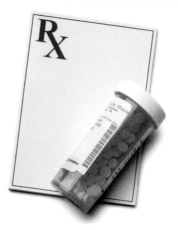

»Faith Life

Does your faith community have Sunday school programs? Today consider starting a Sunday school program that is centered on the wellness journey. Encourage other members of your faith community to live wellness-oriented lives.

»Medical

Remember that medication is not a magical pill. When your physician writes a prescription for a medication, ask questions about what lifestyle changes you should be making along with the medication to be healthier.

»Movement

Today before you eat dinner, do some cardio exercise. Go for a walk, jog in place for five minutes, or do thirty jumping jacks. Exercising before eating will make you feel healthier and will in turn motivate you to eat healthier.

{ We need to be reminded that we are not alone on the journey. }

»Work

If there is someone at your work who shares your particular lunchtime and perhaps is interested in eating healthy meals, adopt that person as a lunch buddy. Take turns bringing in new, healthy dishes to try.

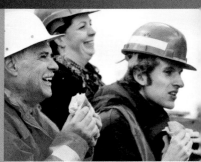

»Emotional

When we feel alone, we can become despondent, and that despondency can halt our progress on the wellness journey. Today spend five minutes writing about the many ways in which you are not alone.

»Family and Friends

Your family and friends can be of great support, but seeking support from people going through an experience similar to yours can also be good. Support groups exist at gyms and wellness centers as well as online. Find a group that you can belong to.

»Nutrition

No matter how much you want to lose weight, do not start a fad diet. While they may help you lose weight, fad diets generally do not promote overall wellness. You will be better off with long-term lifestyle changes.

"My command is this: Love each other as I have loved you. Greater love has no one than this: to lay down one's life for one's friends. You are my friends if you do what I command. . . . You did not choose me, but I chose you and appointed you so that you might go and bear fruit—fruit that will last. . . . This is my command: Love each other."

JOHN 15:12–17

Evening Wrap-Up

As you continue on this journey,

keep in mind that you are loved deeply by Jesus Christ who laid down His life so that we might live. But as we bask in the light of Christ's love, we are also called to live in community, to support one another, and to "bear fruit that will last." Wellness is fruit that will last.

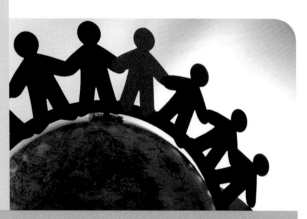

Living Lord, thank You for loving me. Give me the strength to continue on this journey and to encourage others who are also on the journey. In Your holy name, Amen.

Morning Reflection

Today is Day 40—congratulations! You have made it forty days! Over the past six weeks, you have gained the skills necessary to continue on your journey toward wellness. Setbacks will probably happen from time to time, but in the last six weeks, you have set up a foundation that you can return to when needed. The journey to wellness may take you to unexpected places, but wherever wellness takes you, it is sure to lead to a fuller and more abundant life.

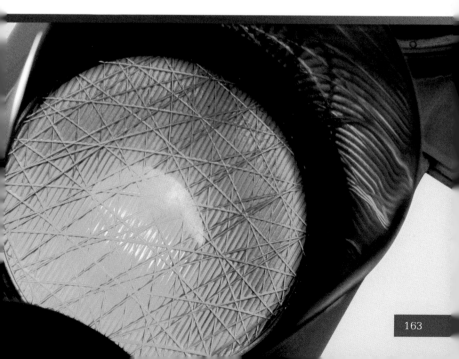

» Faith Life

What does abundant life mean to you? We are told that Jesus came so that we might have life, and life in abundance. What might that mean for you?

» Medical

If you change health care providers, try to get to know them while you are healthy. It is much easier for doctors to treat you when they know what "healthy you" is like.

» Movement

In celebration of life in abundance, put on some music and dance today. Bounce around, get your heart rate up, and don't forget to use your arms!

» Work

If you need to go out to lunch for work, ask for a "to go" box to bring home some of your food. If the portions are larger than what is healthy (as is the case at most restaurants), put half of your order in the box before you eat.

» Emotional

Today try to rest. When we are tired, overworked, and sleep deprived, our body responds to stressors, causing us to hang on to weight and generally feel icky. Even if you only manage to take a twenty-minute nap, it will help you to feel better.

» Family and Friends

Today prepare a meal for your friends and family that you have never pre-pared before. Get your guests to help you prepare the meal, chopping vegetables or stirring the pot as things cook.

» Nutrition

Do not skip breakfast! If you want a change from the usual cereal, try eating leftovers from last night's dinner for breakfast. That'll get you at least a serving of vegetables to start out the day.

Evening Wrap-Up

Remember that God gives us abundant grace through Jesus

Christ and that we are not only given abundant grace in spirit, but in our whole selves and our whole lives. This journey to wellness is about responding appropriately to that abundant grace that Jesus Christ grants us. When we care for ourselves, we are caring for God's creation—the very thing that Jesus came to save.

For if, by the trespass of the one man, death reigned through that one man, how much more will those who receive God's abundant provision of grace and of the gift of righteousness reign in life through the one man, Jesus Christ!

Romans 5:17

Caring God, thank You for walking with me on this journey and for the abundant grace that You give me. Help me today and all days to live my life to abundance in wellness and in grace. In Your holy name, Amen.

Morning Reflection

Now that the forty days are over, today will be a day of review. When we started out this journey, we had to assess where we were in order to set goals for the journey. In a similar manner, we have to assess where we are again so that we can know where we need to go from here. We need to see our successes as well as our setbacks so that we know what we still need to work on.

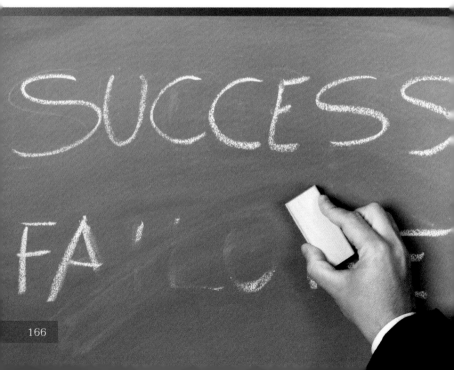

»Faith Life

When we started, you wrote ten words describing your faith life. Again, take five minutes and write ten words describing your faith life now. Then compare the two lists. What has changed? What has stayed the same?

....

....

....

....

....

....

....

....

....

{ We need to see our successes as well as our setbacks. }

»Medical

What are your medical concerns now? Are they significantly different from what they were six weeks ago? Write down your current medical concerns, but do not get rid of your old list of concerns.

....

....

....

....

»Movement

Go for a walk today, and walk as far as you can walk. How far could you walk the first time you did this? Can you feel the improvement in the way your body is reacting to walking?

....

....

....

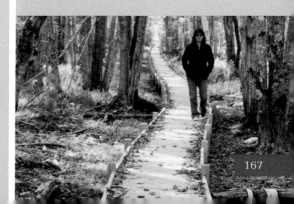

167

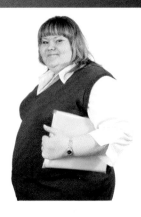

» Work

What has changed about your work environment? Are you drinking more water? Are you eating healthier snacks? Are you getting a little exercise throughout the day?

» Emotional

What has changed in your emotional wellness? Take a look at your emotional highs and lows from Week 2. Do you still have similar highs and lows, or has your overall emotional pattern changed a bit?

» Family and Friends

What have your family and friends thought about your journey? Can they see a difference in you? Take a moment today and ask one or two of them.

» Nutrition

In the first week, you made a list of the foods that you like to eat. Can you expand that list any after six weeks? In particular, can you include more healthy meals on that list?

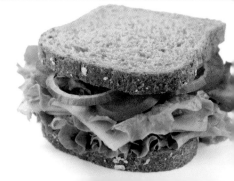

Evening Wrap-Up

The last six weeks have been challenging in a variety of ways. You have been asked to try vastly new things, from food to exercises. You have been asked to step outside your comfort zone and to explore emotions that most of us do not take the time to explore regularly. But the journey—at least this part of the journey—is finished. And you have finished the race. For that, you ought to be very proud and thankful. You have run the race, and God has been running right beside you. Remember as you continue from this point, God runs the race with you. God gives us all strength and endurance when we most need it, and God cheers when we cross the finish line.

I have fought the good fight, I have finished the race, I have kept the faith.

2 TIMOTHY 4:7

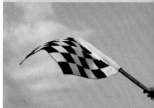

Creator of life, Thank You for the gift of wellness. Help me to continue on this journey with endurance and bravery. In Your holy name, Amen.

Morning Reflection

With the six weeks completed, it can certainly feel as if the journey is over. However, as has been said before, the journey has really only just begun. The journey to wellness is never over. Life will offer us many surprises along the way, and it will be part of the journey to adapt as life happens. Today as we close this chapter on the journey, we look ahead to continue the lessons learned on this journey.

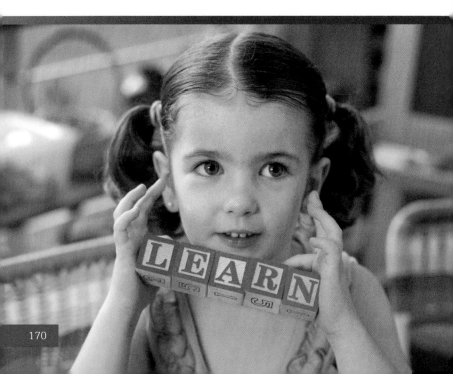

»Faith Life

As you continue on this journey, remember to take time to pray or meditate each day. Prayer and meditation can keep you connected to your purpose and your anchor.

»Medical

Take all medication exactly as prescribed, and do not be afraid to talk to your doctor about anything. The best way to stay medically healthy is to have open communication with your physician.

»Movement

Move everywhere. Find ways to add a few steps to your day in everything you do. A great goal would be to add 200 steps to each day, which will help your body to burn calories more efficiently each day.

{ The journey to wellness is never over. }

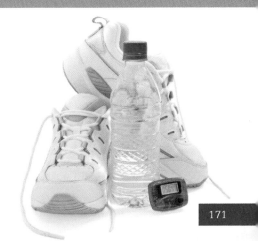

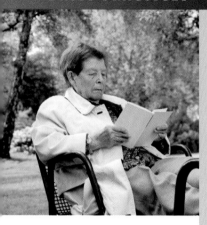

»Work

Try to find time in your day to exercise even a little bit. It will help break up the monotony of the day and will help you to add a few steps. Also, avoid office junk food. Instead, opt for healthy snacks and lunches.

»Emotional

Find and remember ways that you can relieve stress. Take a hot bath, go for a walk, or read a book. Just find something that works for you and do it every day. The more you relieve your stress, the better you will feel and the healthier you will become.

»Family and Friends

Remember that your family and friends are your support system. When you are struggling, do not be afraid to lean on them for support, and when you have succeeded, do not be afraid to celebrate with them.

»Nutrition

Make your calories count. Enjoy all of the wonderful colors and flavors of God's creation as you prepare meals using whole grains, a variety of fruits and vegetables, and lean meats—but let yourself splurge on occasion!

Evening Wrap-Up

It has been a long journey to this point, but you have been given many tools to continue on your way. You will find other tools to add to your toolbox, and you will have setbacks. But remember that God walks with you, and God can grant you peace, even when you have a difficult time finding it for yourself.

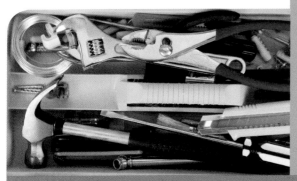

Finally, brothers and sisters, whatever is true, whatever is noble, whatever is right, whatever is pure, whatever is lovely, whatever is admirable— if anything is excellent or praiseworthy— think about such things. Whatever you have learned or received or heard from me, or seen in me— put it into practice. And the God of peace will be with you.

PHILIPPIANS 4:8–9

God of health and healing, be with me as I continue on this journey. Help me to remember the things I have learned, and help me to continue learning. I will continue to strive to honor my body and my whole self, Your creation. In Your holy name, Amen.

Recommended Reading and Resources

Websites
Church Health Reader, www.chreader.org. Church Health Reader is the online and print publication of the Church Health Center. Church Health Reader provides resources for you and your church to become healthier in body and spirit. It offers interviews with leaders and thinkers, tips and advice on running effective ministries, and practical suggestions for individuals and churches. The print version is published four times a year and is available through yearly subscription or online at www.chreader.org

Books
Regaining the Power of Youth at Any Age by Kenneth H. Cooper. This book features a scientifically based program that will guide you to a higher level of physical and mental fitness than you may have believed possible to attain.

What to Eat by Marion Nestle. Nestle walks readers through every super-market section—produce, meat, fish, dairy, packaged foods, bottled waters, and more—decoding labels and clarifying nutritional and other claims (in supermarket-speak, for example, "fresh" means most likely to spoil first, not recently picked or prepared), and in so doing explores issues such as the effects of food production on our environment, the way pricing works, and additives and their effect on nutrition.

The Inner Game of Stress: Outsmart Life's Challenges and Fulfill Your Potential by W. Timothy Gallwey. Renowned sports psychology expert W. Timothy Gallwey teams up with two esteemed physicians to offer a unique and em-powering guide to mental health in today's volatile world. *The Inner Game of Stress* applies the trusted principles of Gallwey's wildly popular Inner Game series, which have helped athletes the world over, to the manage-ment of everyday stress—personal, professional, financial, physical—and shows us how to access our inner resources to maintain stability and achieve success.

Your Child's Weight: Helping without Harming by Ellyn Satter. As much about parenting as feeding, this latest release from renowned childhood feeding expert Ellyn Satter considers the overweight child issue in a new way. Combining scientific research with inspiring anecdotes from her decades of clinical practice, Satter challenges the conventional belief that parents must get overweight children to eat less and exercise more.

Mindless Eating: Why We Eat More Than We Think by Brian Wansink. In this illuminating and groundbreaking new book, food psychologist Brian Wansink shows why you may not realize how much you're eating, what you're eating—or why you're even eating at all.

Change or Die: The Three Keys to Change at Work and in Life by Alan Deutschman. A powerful book with universal appeal, *Change or Die* deconstructs and debunks age-old myths about change and empowers us with three critical keys—relate, repeat, and reframe—to help us make important positive changes in our lives. Explaining breakthrough research and progressive ideas from a wide selection of leaders in medicine, science, and business, Deutschman demonstrates how anyone can achieve lasting, revolutionary changes that are positive, attainable, and absolutely vital.

Family Health, Nutrition and Fitness by Paul C. Reisser. This book will help you take an active role in improving the health and well-being of you and your family by offering authoritative and current medical information in a convenient, easy-to-understand format. Taking a balanced, commonsense approach to the issue of health and wellness, this indispensable guide delivers an encouraging perspective with helpful reference sections.

40 Days to Better Living

A series of practical books
dealing with specific health issues

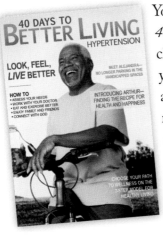

You want to feel better—and *40 Days to Better Living* provides clear, manageable steps to get you there through life-changing attitudes and actions. If you're ready to live better, select one or more elements of the Seven-Step Model for Healthy Living—Faith Life, Medical, Movement, Work, Emotional, Family and Friends, and Nutrition—and follow the forty-day plan to improve your life, just a bit, day by day. With plenty of practical advice, biblical encouragement, and stories of real people who have taken the same journey, this may be the most important book you read this year!

Bimonthly release schedule, beginning July 2011.

Titles to include:

Optimal Health / Hypertension / Depression / Smoking Cessation / Weight Management / Stress Management / Aging / Addiction / Diabetes / Anxiety / Caregiving

Available wherever Christian books are sold.